Dreas Reyneke is celebra
bution to the art and ⸱   ⸱⸱⸱⸱⸱⸱⸱ ⸱⸱⸱⸱⸱⸱⸱. A
former dancer with the Ballet Rambert, he taught at
the first pilates studio to open in London, and in 1973
he opened his Body Conditioning Studio in Notting
Hill, where he developed his pilates-based training
method. His clientele includes stars past and present
from dance, theatre, television, and cinema, and some
great names in sport, literature, and journalism. At the
beginning of the year 2000 his studio was voted one
of the best pilates studios in London by the city's
daily newspaper, the *Evening Standard*, and by leading
international style magazines. His book *Ultimate
Pilates*, presenting his unique exercise system, is to be
published early in 2002.

Helen Varley is a journalist and author whose first edi-
torial venture into the world of aviation was during
the 1980s as general editor and major contributor to
the first popular guide to air travel and airports, *The
Flier's Handbook*. During the 1980s she founded and
developed the *Time Out* series of guides to London
life, and *Time Out* travel guides. In the early 1990s she
wrote *Weekends Across the Channel* to celebrate the
opening of the Channel Tunnel. She continues to write
widely in the fields of travel, medicine and healing.

MEDICAL CONSULTANT

Dr Maria Stack is well known in the specialized field of aviation medicine as one of the few women Authorised Medical Examiners for the Civil Aviation Authority, the UK's regulatory body for aviation. In addition to her work in assessing pilots' health, she runs the Farnborough International Travel and Aviation Clinic at Farnborough Airport near London, providing health care to corporate clients and to individual travellers. Before specializing in aviation medicine, Dr Stack had a distinguished medical career in the fields of children's and women's health. She maintains a busy schedule of broadcasting and media work to publicize issues central to health: as a medical contributor and panellist on local radio stations, as preventive health specialist in the local press, and as a contributor to the Sky Medical Channel and Meridian TV on topical health issues. Contact her website, www.fitac2000.com, for information on economy class syndrome, immunizations, malaria prevention, air travel during pregnancy, and many other aspects of air travel and health.

In-Flight Fitness

DREAS REYNEKE

with Helen Varley

ORION

An Orion Paperback
First published in Great Britain in 2001 by
Orion Books Ltd,
Orion House, 5 Upper St Martin's Lane,
London WC2H 9EA

A CIP catalogue record for this book
is available from the British Library.

ISBN: 0 75284 458 X

Printed and bound in Great Britain by
The Guernsey Press Co. Ltd, Guernsey, C.I.

CONTENTS

INTRODUCTION
You Must Be Fit to Fly

Flying used to be the cool way to travel, luxurious and glamorous, and a seat in economy class was half the fun of going on holiday. But deregulation and competition, soaring fuel costs, booming passenger payloads, and overcrowded airports have reduced even first-class travel to a test of stamina. An economy-class seat from Tokyo to New York or Amsterdam to Manila may now be the most uncomfortable and potentially unhealthy mode of transport.

These days, you need to be fit to fly, because high-capacity airliners are carrying more passengers higher and further than ever before. The new Boeing 777 can fly at 13,100 metres (43,000 feet), and Boeing's proposed subsonic cruiser will cruise at 13,700 metres (45,000 feet). Sitting in the pressurized cabin of a high-flying jet is roughly equivalent to standing on top of Mount St Helens in Washington State, USA, where the air is thin and very dry. It can be hard to breathe, especially if you are very young, or getting on in years, or not as fit as you might be. Passengers with breathing problems need extra oxygen.

In-flight exercising

A year ago the idea of exercising in-flight would have astonished most airline passengers, but as this book goes to press the larger airlines are publishing leg exercises in their in-flight magazines, and showing exercise videos to passengers on long-haul flights. What has brought this change about is the publicity surrounding 'economy class syndrome', the health scare story currently in the news. In fact it affects first-class and business-class passengers as well as those in the economy cabin. Its medical name is deep-vein thrombosis, because blood clots develop in the deep veins of the legs, and these can stop the blood circulation, and may break away to block blood flow to the lungs and other major organs. Prolonged inactivity owing to being confined in a cramped economy seat on a long-haul flight has recently been identified as a likely cause.

Keeping the blood moving by walking up and down the cabin and stretching the feet and legs is said to be the best way to prevent this illness. But how much walking is possible in a busy economy-class cabin, and how effective can a few foot stretches be? The focus of this book is a set of exercises designed to be done seated in an economy-class cabin. They work the muscles of the feet and calves, thighs and even the hips, keeping the blood moving and distributing oxygen to the brain and body tissues.

Sitting in a crowded cabin for many hours on a long flight with scarcely a chance to move can cause other health problems in addition to blood clots. Muscle and joint stiffness, tension in neck and shoulders, lower-back pain, and shallow breathing which causes palpitations, headaches, and breathlessness are common health consequences of long-haul travel. The exercise programmes in Chapter 4 include self-massage and stretching, breathing and relaxation techniques designed to remedy and to prevent these health effects.

Endurance vs. Health

New-generation jetliners are breaking long-distance records, and we may be at the point, as one aviation journalist wrote recently, 'when the endurance of the aircraft could exceed the endurance of the passenger'. He was writing about designing comfortable seats for business jets capable of flying fourteen-hour trips. Meanwhile, airlines are buying in a new generation of monster passenger jets and planning to fly them non-stop from London to Sydney. A flight of 16–18 hours in an economy seat just 44 centimetres (17.5 inches) wide, with a miserly pitch of perhaps 74 centimetres (29 inches) from the cushion you sit back against to the back of the seat in front, could be a special, 21st-century torture.

Some of the health effects of long-haul air travel have come to light only since the 1990s. Little research has been done and information is available mainly to doctors working in what is an increasingly specialized field. British GPs and other primary care doctors often have only minimal training in aviation medicine. And apart from an occasional article in travel magazines, passengers get little information other than scare stories in the press.

In this book we try to close the gap. We look at what is known about how and why blood clots develop in the leg veins and we explain what, in addition to exercise, you can do to prevent them. We explore the whole range of illnesses associated with flying, from asthma to earache and fainting to jet lag, and explain their causes, how they are treated, and what you can do to prevent them. An aircraft cabin is an abnormal environment for the human body, so that small complaints you would normally dismiss, such as head colds and sinus problems, can have serious effects when descending from 10,700 metres (35,000 feet). Passengers need to be fully informed to be able to assess their fitness to fly.

Take control

Flying affects the mind and body, but there are many things you can do to help yourself avoid its ill-effects. Every body is different and responds in an individual way to treatments and remedies. The expert advice of our Medical Consultant, Dr Maria Stack, a specialist in aviation medicine, is given for the treatment of every aviation illness. And to her suggestions we add remedies from alternative therapists working in different fields, plus common-sense measures contributed by a few frequent fliers who have worked out their own solutions to the adverse health effects of flying. The simplest, most obvious measures can often prevent harmful physical and mental reactions.

An aircraft cruising 10.5 kilometres (7 miles) high is an unnatural environment, and we survive only because complex aircraft systems supply air and air pressure, heat and water. These systems are not faultless, and there is much controversy about the cabin's internal air pressure, the use of recirculated, filtered air, and antiquated water systems. In Chapters 5, 6 and 7 we summarize the main points of how these life-support systems work, the arguments for and against retaining them, and anything that is known about their effects, if any, on health. Passengers generally feel they have no voice in the debates that rage over these important issues, so we suggest action you can take to lobby airlines, governing bodies and passenger support groups to make your opinions known.

Keeping a perspective

Through these arguments and controversies it is essential to maintain a perspective. Passenger comfort is important and passenger health is still more so, but safety is paramount. And aircraft safety is costly. Deregulation began at a time of massive expansion in air travel, and the traveller benefited, flying further and faster in new generations of jets for steadily falling ticket prices. However, faced with rising fuel prices, newly competitive airlines had to find ways of cutting costs, and the area they found to cut was in economy class. The economics of airline pricing are complex, but roughly summarized, the first-class and business-class seats account for some 70–80 per cent of airline revenue. More and more people are flying at cut or discounted prices (how many 'air miles' are given away each year?). Far more people want the cheapest possible seats than want to pay first- or business-class prices, yet economy seats account for only 20–30 per cent of revenue. The more seats an airline can cram into economy class, the more tickets it can sell, and the higher its profits.

Yet although airlines are heavily criticized for being motivated to maximize profits more than passenger comfort and health, it seems that their profits are not excessive. During the 1990s more than 100 airlines went bankrupt, and at the end of the decade Pat Hanlon, Senior Lecturer at Birmingham University's Business School, wrote in his book *Global Airlines*, 'The industry may have achieved high rates of growth, but this has not been accompanied by high rates of profitability, quite the opposite. Airline profit margins have been well below average compared with firms in other industries, and in some years there have been some very heavy losses indeed.'

Every year 1,200 scheduled airlines fly 1.5 billion passengers to their destinations with an admirable safety record. The cost of maintaining that record and of improving passenger health and comfort in the ways suggested in this book will be shouldered by the airlines. To satisfy passengers' rising standards of health and safety, airlines are faced with the need to raise ticket prices.

Shop around

'Cheapest flights' are what the cut-price ticket websites on the Internet advertise. But if passengers want airlines to carry them in safety and comfort, ensuring that they reach their destination in the same state of health as when they left home, there need to be 'safe-flight ticket' websites offering maximum health and comfort. The young and the very fit can withstand a flight in economy class with minimal ill-effects. Older people, pregnant women and nursing mothers, children, and people with illnesses, especially those in the risk categories for developing blood clots, need to think about upgrading.

Some airlines are already upgrading, offering 'premium economy' with larger, more comfortable seats and more leg room. Significantly more of us upgrading to premium economy and business class would eventually change the economics of airline pricing. Imagine an Airbus with a tiny economy-class cabin at the back and a spacious premium-class cabin with roomy seats that recline down into beds for overnight flights. Imagine the demise of first class, with premium-economy-only Boeings on long-haul routes, with passengers paying higher but affordable prices for the extra space and comfort.

'Take control' is the theme of this book, and the consumer has the power to do so. Don't just book the cheapest ticket, shop around for cabin health and comfort.

CHAPTER ONE
Keeping Healthy and Fit In-Flight

'My left foot is obstructed by a metal box beneath my seat, my elbows are jogging my neighbour, and I can't stand up without hitting the air vents. My knees are touching the seat in front, and when it reclines back it presses down on my left knee ...' reported one frequent flier who tested our exercises in economy class. This air traveller was 5 feet 10 inches – just over 1.75 metres – and tall people suffer horrendously from the restricted space in economy class.

Wedging yourself into a tight seat for a short-haul flight from London to Glasgow, or Paris to Nice will make you stiff and uncomfortable, but you are unlikely to suffer any permanent damage. On a longer journey of four hours or more it can cause serious health problems. The crowded seating arrangements in the main cabins of long-distance passenger jets made 'economy class syndrome' the turn-of-the-millennium media buzzphrase. It is the popular name for what medical people call deep-vein thrombosis (DVT), because blood clots develop in the deep veins of the legs.

DVT affects one person in every 1,000 aged over sixty-five and one person in every 10,000 aged under sixty-five, whether they fly or drive, or sit in economy- or first-class seats. But physicians believe that sitting immobile for hours in cramped economy-class seats encourages blood clots to form in the leg veins. Too few studies have been carried out for reliable figures to be available, but it is estimated that between one person in ten and one in twenty is likely to develop blood clots – so as many as fifteen people on a 260-scater jet may be at risk. Chapter 2 explains deep-vein thrombosis as it affects air travellers, giving the results of the latest research, explaining who is most at risk, its symptoms and its long-term effects, and suggesting action you can take to prevent it affecting you.

Back strain is another economy class syndrome. In fact, many more passengers who travel in economy class suffer with back problems than with deep-vein thrombosis. Sitting in a cramped position without being able to move your legs puts great strain on your back. If you have back trouble, the stress of a long-haul flight can make it worse. If you are reading this book just before or on a long-haul flight, turn to Chapter 3 now. It explores various different ways to reduce the strain and make your back feel more comfortable during a long flight.

Media focus on deep-vein thrombosis, the effects on health of cabin pressurization, and the question of cabin air quality may lead airlines and aircraft manufacturers to address these issues and improve many aspects of passenger health and comfort in coming years. But because the human body was designed to live at sea level and to move around constantly, sitting for long periods in an aircraft 10,700 metres (35,000 feet) up and travelling at 1,000 k.p.h. (600 m.p.h.) is always going to bring health problems. This chapter looks at things you can do in-flight and before you fly to ensure a healthier and more enjoyable journey.

Action!

If you are reading this book on a long-haul flight, sitting in economy class, what can you do *now* to protect your health and improve your comfort? Try some of these measures before reading any further:

■ **If you are 1.75 metres (5 feet 9 inches) or taller,** you may be experiencing real discomfort. Because you have so little room for your legs, you fall into the 'at-risk' category for developing blood clots in your leg veins. Every aircraft has a few seats in economy class with more space in front for passengers' legs, some near emergency exits. Some airlines reserve these seats for tall passengers. (Qantas will often take advance bookings for these seats on long-haul routes). Call a flight attendant over *now*, show how cramped your legs are, and:

- Ask if you can be upgraded to a spare seat in business class, or:
- Ask if you can be moved to a seat with more leg room.

■ **If you are 1.5 metres (5 feet) or shorter,** you may find that when you sit back in your seat, your feet do not reach the floor. This might mean that the cushion is pressed hard against the seat edge, compressing veins in your legs, which puts you in the 'at-risk' category for developing blood clots in your leg veins. You need to take action. Find something you can rest your feet on to raise your knees away from the edge of the cushion. If you can put a bag on the floor, use that. If not, call a flight attendant over *now*, demonstrate the problem, and:

● Ask to be upgraded to a seat with a footrest, or:
● Ask the flight attendant to find something you can rest your feet on.

■ **Action for everyone** (*especially* if you are middle-aged or elderly, have varicose veins or a history of leg swelling or blood clots, or you are a woman on the contraceptive pill, or HRT, or if you are pregnant). The following measures will help prevent blood clots from forming, and the exercises will ease stress on your lower back:

● Ask for still bottled water, and drink a glass every hour or so. (Do not substitute with alcoholic or carbonated soft drinks, coffee or tea – all these drinks are dehydrating.)
● Ask if compression socks are supplied or sold on board the aircraft. If so, buy a pair in your size and wear them during the trip.
● Ask if the airline supplies exercise mats. Emirates is one airline to have ordered abundant supplies of the Airogym (see page 49) for its passengers to use on board, and others may follow. An exercise mat increases the effectiveness of exercising while sitting in a cabin seat.
● Turn to page 90-94 and do the circulation-boosting exercises now, and repeat them once an hour while you are awake, for the duration of the trip.
● Every four hours, work through the complete programme of exercises on pages 95–111.

Make yourself comfortable

Only on a long-haul flight would you sit, scarcely moving, for eight hours or more. You are in an extreme situation and your comfort and health are interlinked. Normally, you pay little attention if you feel slightly hot, because you can easily move into a cooler environment, or rest. But physical discomforts often have a knock-on effect when you are airborne. For instance, heat makes you perspire, and in time that will dehydrate you. Dehydration thickens the blood and so encourages the formation of blood clots. It dries the mucous lining of your nose and throat, reducing their power to fight infection, so you become more susceptible to colds and throat infections.

Take time now to think about how comfortable you are. Aspects of flying that often make people feel uncomfortable, such as low air pressure and dehydration, are explored in Chapters 5 and 6, which list many things you can do to make yourself feel more comfortable. Here are a few actions to take early in the flight:

■ **How are you dressed?** Ideally on a long air journey you need to wear comfortable, loose-fitting clothes. If you rushed from work to the aircraft, you may be in rather formal work clothes. Do you have anything in your hand luggage you can change into? If not:

● Loosen a tight belt and collar.
● If you are wearing socks or support hose with elastic tops that grip at the knee or the thigh, roll them down or take them off. On a long flight they will

restrict the blood circulation to your legs and that can encourage blood clots.

- Are you too warm? If you can, peel off outer layers such as jackets and jerseys, and stow them in the overhead locker. Ask for a drink of refrigerated water to reduce your body heat.
- Are you too cold? Dress in layers for a long air trip so you can don an extra t-shirt or a jumper if you feel cold. You need to keep warm because when you fly, stress may reduce your natural resistance to colds and infections. Look after yourself: ask a flight attendant for a blanket and a hot drink.
- How do your feet feel? It is best to take a pair of soft, light shoes to wear on the aircraft. On a long flight your feet and ankles usually swell a little because the circulating blood tends to stagnate there. Can you take your shoes off and rest your feet on a magazine?

Stress and fatigue

Preparing to travel, getting to the airport, and nervousness about flying are stressful, and this is why fatigue often sets in once a flight is under way. If a rush to board the flight has left you feeling limp, now is the time to review your situation.

- When did you last eat? If you have been fuelling your energy with coffees you are probably mildly dehydrated, and dehydration causes fatigue. Drink a glass or two of still water and in about ten minutes you will begin to feel better. A light meal will revive and relax you if you have not eaten. Do not eat salty snacks, such as crisps, or chocolate because they are dehydrating.

- If you intend to nap after you have eaten, leave your seat beforehand and exercise your legs by walking along the aisle of the aircraft. If the aisle is too crowded, at least visit the washroom as soon as you can and use the opportunity to stretch your legs and exercise your feet. Sleeping in cramped seating may be linked with the development of blood clots, so before sleeping do all the things recommended on pages 78-80.

- If you find it difficult to relax and impossible to sleep, make yourself as comfortable as you can, do the breathing and stretching and the relaxation exercises in Chapter 4, then read or watch a video. If you are a business traveller, plan a work-free hour or two. Rest is a good substitute for sleep, so exercise and follow with relaxation two or three times on a long flight.

The effects of stress

If you are a frequent flier, plan ways of minimizing stress on future trips. Stress is repeated or prolonged mental turmoil, and although its effects on health may often be greatly exaggerated, the core facts remain. The body responds with muscular tension and the release of excess adrenaline and other hormones into the blood, and these effects can undermine the immune system. When you travel, this makes you susceptible to infection by disease-causing bacteria and viruses that transmit colds and flu. Here are a few measures you can take to reduce the stress and anxiety of travelling:

- Try to arrange things so you have time to exercise and relax the day before the flight. The exercises in Chapter 4 are designed to defuse stress. Do them to help yourself sleep well.

- Take at least 30mg of vitamin B-complex for two to three days before flying.

- Massage is a great stress-reliever, so fit in a massage some time before your flight. Some airlines make massage available in-flight to first-class passengers, while others have massage facilities in the first-class departure lounge in the airport, so make the most of them if you have a first-class ticket.

- Give yourself plenty of time to get to the airport, taking the most reliable means of transport, not necessarily the fastest. Worrying about whether you can get through the traffic is stressful. It may be better to take a train.

- If you are thinking of using the airport's long-term car park, check out in advance how to get from parked car to check-in. The long-term car park is often a long way from the airport and it can take you more than an hour to reach the air terminal. Arriving at the check-in desk in a panic is a common cause of stress among frequent business travellers. It may be better to travel by bus, train, underground, or taxi, or hire a car.

- Accept that you may have to queue in a crowded airport to check in. Do not get ruffled. Take a book or music to listen to while standing in line. Enjoy the busy scene around you. Chat with people in the line.
- If your flight is delayed, do not let frustration get the better of you. Telephone to rearrange your schedule, then try to use the time enjoyably. Explore the airport. Watch the maintenance crew breaking records to get your grounded flight into the air. There may be an observation balcony overlooking the airfield. London's Heathrow has a multidenomi-national chapel with an open-air garden, where anyone can go for peace and quiet. In some British airports economy-class passengers can pay a small fee to sit and wait in a comfortable passenger lounge.
- If the air terminal is uncomfortable and there is nothing to do, put your luggage in a locker and walk around, climb stairs, do the exercises on pages 95–111. Then find an empty seat and do the breathing and relaxation exercises on pages 111–116.
- A healthy diet high in wholegrain cereals, fruit and vegetables and low in refined carbohydrates and caffeine is thought to benefit the immune system.
- Alternative therapists recommend echinacea, available as drops to take in water or as capsules.

Jet lag

On the flight to a distant destination you can do a lot to minimize the effects of jet lag – the tiredness and disorientation you experience when you travel across several time zones. Most of the body's many internal systems run to a 24-hour clock, and every activity from falling asleep and waking up to the release of hormones and the digestion and elimination of food keep time with it. The pineal gland deep in the brain governs the body's 24-hour activity cycles through hormones it releases. Crossing time zones upsets their release pattern and puts all the body's cycles out of synch.

Jet lag is worse when you fly eastwards, because you gain time. The best solution is to travel on a flight leaving in the early evening with one of the larger airlines and book a business-class seat that converts into a flat bed. It is well worth while paying extra to sleep through the night, because sleeping in a cramped economy-class seat encourages blood clots to develop. Alternatives are to travel through the day, taking an early flight, and to sleep late or nap before the flight. If you fly westwards, stay awake until the bedtime at your destination to re-establish a new body rhythm as quickly as possible. Jet lag can be a serious problem for frequent business fliers, who need to search for a workable solution that enables them to get as much sleep in every twenty-four hours as in a normal 24-hour period at home.

Many remedies have been suggested and marketed to combat jet lag. The following have proved the most effective, but people react very differently to jet lag and you need to read around the subject, try out different remedies, and find what works for you.

Before you go:

- Build up a reserve by getting as much sleep as you can during the week before the flight.
- Work on a regular pre-sleep routine, such as the stretching–breathing–relaxation exercises in Chapter 4.
- If you can, try to fly by day and arrive at night.

During the flight:

- Act as if you are there: work out what are normal mealtimes and sleeping times at your destination and eat and sleep as close as you can to those times in-flight. If possible, try to do the same for a day or two before your trip.
- Alternative therapists recommend vitamin B-complex supplements, anti-oxidants, and No-Jet-Lag homeopathic tablets, available from homeopathic chemists and from airline shops at airports. Check the website (see page 195) for more information and details of stockists world-wide.
- Melatonin is widely agreed to be effective in preventing jet lag and reducing its symptoms. It is the hormone produced by the pineal gland, which regulates the sleep-wake cycle. Melatonin can be bought as tablets from health stores in the USA and other countries. Reliable research suggests that less than 1mg taken close to midnight in your destination country the day before you arrive, and for the next two or three days, helps your body clock to adjust fairly painlessly to the new regime. However, a word

of warning: melatonin is banned in the UK since it may have harmful long-term effects. For this same reason, it must not be taken every day, women who might be or are pregnant or nursing should not take it, and it must not be given to children.

When you arrive:

- Whenever you feel sleepy and circumstances allow, sleep or nap.
- Do not go to bed hungry, but do not eat or drink close to bedtime.
- If you wake before morning and cannot get back to sleep within half an hour, get out of bed and do something that will help you relax. Do not drink alcohol, cola, caffeinated tea or coffee, or eat or drink chocolate, which contains caffeine. Go back to bed when you feel tired enough to sleep even for just a short time.
- A nap of up to forty-five minutes before an important event will restore your alertness and performance.
- Spend as much daylight time as you can out of doors. Sunlight is believed to slow or stop the body clock, making it easier to adjust to new time schedules.
- Total relaxation after a long international flight and then twice a day for ten minutes is the hatha yoga way of combating jet lag. Lie on a mat on the floor with your head in line with your body, the lower part of the back of your head touching the floor. Lift your head slightly and shake it very gently. Stretch

your ankles and let your feet fall outwards. Lift your arms a little and let them fall back on to the mat, palms facing up. Then close your eyes and breathe gently and rhythmically through your nose, concentrating on relaxing each part of your body in turn, beginning with your toes. If you cannot lie down, find a quiet spot and do the exercise while sitting.

Airsickness

If you feel nauseous in-flight, do not immediately blame motion sickness. It is more common among people travelling on ships than in the air. You may get indigestion because you cannot walk around after an in-flight meal. Ask a flight attendant for an indigestion tablet and take it with water. If you can, walk along the aisle for a while. Sit back in your seat and breathe in and out steadily for a few minutes, because slight nausea can be caused by shallow breathing, which reduces blood oxygen levels (see pages 121–2). Lack of food and water combined with stress can make you feel nauseous, so do not neglect to eat and drink while flying.

Motion sickness occurs because confusing signals about position and orientation are sent from the ears, where the organs of balance are located, and from the eyes to the brain. Here are a few remedies:
- Ask a flight attendant to find you a seat close to the centre of the cabin where any pitching and rolling is minimal.
- Focus your eyes on some distant object which is

fixed and horizontal. Do not read or watch a video.

- Travel sickness tablets for long journeys contain sedative antihistamine drugs, such as Promethazine, and anticholinergic drugs, which act on the nerves, such as Hyoscine. They are more or less effective in different individuals, so you will need to consult a pharmacist and try out different travel sickness tablets until you find one that works. You normally take them two hours or one hour before the flight (check the pack). They have side-effects, so do not overdose, or drink alcohol or drive on the day you take one. They can cause blurred vision and a degree of dehydration.

- Alternative therapists recommend taking teabags of ginger tea and asking for hot water, or suspending four drops of essential oils of peppermint and ginger in a carrier lotion and packing it in your hand luggage to sniff if you feel nauseous.

- If you suffer from severe motion sickness, you should consult a physician to try to find a remedy. In-flight, keep drinking water so that you do not become dehydrated.

Are you fit to fly?

It is important to maintain perspective and to bear in mind that thousands of people fly long-distance with no ill-effects. Most passengers need only take common-sense action to keep comfortable and prevent back strain and the formation of blood clots.

Categories of people listed below are more at risk, however, and need to make more preparation for long air trips. People with certain medical conditions need to consult a physician and make special arrangements before booking a ticket. They are listed in the appendix on page 187.

Mothers and children

Radiation risk

Women who might be pregnant should consider that aircraft fly at altitudes where radiation from the sun is at a much higher level than at sea level. The maximum recommended total exposure to the abdomen during pregnancy is 1 milliSievert per year (mSv: Sieverts are a measure of the amount of radiation absorbed and the damage that dose can do to the body). As a guide, Concorde flies much higher than subsonic jet airliners and receives almost twice as much radiation, and its air crew receive 2–3 mSv in one year of regular flying. Were Concorde to fly over the Poles, where radiation levels are higher than towards the Equator, on every trip for one year, cabin crew would receive an average 6 mSv.

In the light of these averages, women flight crew who might be pregnant may be allocated non-flying duties. European airlines are currently monitoring the exposure levels experienced by staff, so more information may soon be available. However, a passenger flying only a few times a year will not receive enough radiation to affect the foetus. Despite this reassurance, women who might be pregnant may wish to consider that the developing embryo is more at risk from radiation than later, when it is more developed, and decide not to fly until after the fifth week of pregnancy.

If you have had fertilization treatment, if you are pregnant for the first time, or if you have a tendency to miscarry early in pregnancy, it is sensible not to fly long-haul during the first trimester. Some airlines refuse to carry women after the twenty-eighth week of pregnancy because of the risk of premature labour. However, it is safe to fly between the fifth and the twenty-eighth weeks, as long as you take the following precautions:

- During pregnancy the risk of developing blood clots increases significantly. It is important to take all the precautions against developing blood clots in the leg veins listed on pages 12–13 and in Chapter 2. However, do not take aspirin without consulting an obstetrician.

- Your lower back comes under increasing strain as your pregnancy advances, so read Chapter 3 and take all the precautions you can against back strain and sprain. In addition, maternity belts sold by the Back Shop (see page 195) and surgical equipment suppliers are recommended for pregnant women to support the back during a long flight.

- Do not take airsickness tablets, inhalants or other remedies without first consulting a physician.

- Gaviscon tablets are an effective remedy for indigestion and wind problems and are safe to take during pregnancy.

- If you are anaemic, you may need extra oxygen. (This must be requested when booking your ticket and you may be asked to pay for its supply.)
- As your pregnancy advances you may find an economy class seat too small and very uncomfortable. Pay the extra to upgrade to premium economy or business class, where the seats are more roomy and have footrests and back supports.

Children

Little research appears to have been carried out on the effects of long-distance flight on children. However, seating for young children is carefully regulated. Infants and children under the age of two need to be in a certified child seat which has to be secured to an aircraft seat. This does not mean that you necessarily have to purchase a separate ticket. Book well in advance, say you are travelling with a young child, and you should be able to book 'basinet space' for a small fee. This is a specially designed air seat secured against a bulkhead (cabin wall) into which the infant is placed and secured with a child restraint. The infant therefore faces the tail of the aircraft – a much safer position than facing forwards if there is turbulence or during emergency braking. Older children must be in their own aircraft seat and restrained with the airline seat belt – you cannot use a child harness – or in a child air seat. You may be able to use your own child safety seat for children aged over two (or weighing more than 18 kilograms, 2.5 stone or 40 pounds), since most are certified for air travel. Check the label. Airlines can be very helpful in arranging child seating, but they have a limited number of child seats on each flight, so it is essential to book well in advance and to make these arrangements when booking.

Here are a few more important points to bear in mind:

- Newborn babies should not fly until at least forty-eight hours after birth, because their lungs are not fully developed and they can suffer oxygen deprivation. Dehydration can adversely affect babies during the first two weeks.
- Babies need to feed or suck something, or be allowed to cry as the aircraft descends. Older children should be given a drink or sweets to suck, or told to swallow repeatedly. Sucking and swallowing are essential to prevent damage to the inner ear during air-pressure changes. Earplugs called earplanes® are now available to relieve inner ear discomfort in children. Buy them from pharmacists.
- Check that older children have something their feet can press down on when they sit back in the cabin seat so that the backs of their knees and calves do not press down on the seat. This encourages blood clots to form; although this is rare in young people, it does occur.

The middle-aged and elderly

The arbitrary age of forty or fifty usually separates younger from older, yet there may be as much difference between fifty-one and eighty-one as there is between twenty-one and fifty-one. If you are in your fifties and healthy, a long-haul flight is unlikely to make you ill. However, it is important to check your fitness to fly if you have any medical condition. Check the list below and take any recommended precautions, and consult your physician before booking.

- The risk of developing deep-vein thrombosis increases with age, so that after forty you move into the at-risk group. Take all the precautions listed in Chapter 2.
- The incidence of back trouble increases with age, because, unless you have kept your back very supple muscles and tendons are less flexible. Take special note of the precautions listed in Chapter 3. Upgrade to a premium economy- or business-class seat.
- Taking one 75 mg aspirin before a flight will help prevent heart attacks and strokes as well as deep-vein thrombosis, but do not take aspirin if you have gastric irritation or an allergy to aspirin.
- Do not fly if you have a cold or bronchial infection. Have a flu injection (in the winter months in temperate zones) before flying to minimize the risk of catching a chest infection at the airport, from another passenger, or at your destination.

Keep moving

Pilots are aware that they must take positive action to overcome the discomforts of flying and stay alert and efficient, and to keep fit to withstand the strains and fatigue of long-distance travel. An aircraft is not like a train or a bus, operating in close-to-normal conditions for the human body. To take a medium- or long-haul trip cocooned in a pressurized cabin full of noise and vibration is to subject the whole body to fairly extreme conditions, however cheap or expensive the seat. Passengers, like pilots, need to prepare and train for a flight, especially if they fly frequently. If you work out regularly in a gym or practise a sport you are in good shape for flying.

If you are reading this while planning a flight, think about getting into shape. A few simple stretching exercises like those below makes your back more flexible and less likely to suffer strain on a long flight. They will also protect you against developing blood clots. Exercise as simple as walking stimulates the production of plasmin, the body's natural anti-clotting protein which dissolves blood clots as they form, preventing them from enlarging.

There is plenty of scope for exercising en route. If your flight is delayed, sitting around the bar drinking coffee is the wrong reaction. Leave your hand luggage in a locker and walk around. Airports offer plenty of walking potential – large expanses of terminal floor and long travelators to stride along, stairs and escalators to walk briskly up and down two or three times.

Also use waiting time on a stopover to stretch your back and your legs, move your body, and walk around. Put some spring into your walk: shuffling to the bar will do no good. The muscles act as a pump, pressing on the leg veins to send the blood shooting upwards. Energetic, springy walking steps achieve this: heel to the ground, then the toes, heel, then toes, alternately contracting and relaxing each group of leg muscles.

Here is a short programme of daily exercises to get you into training. Start one week before your flight:

Walking practice
- Go for a fifteen-minute walk every day: stride out, stretching your legs. Swing your arms as you go.

Back roll

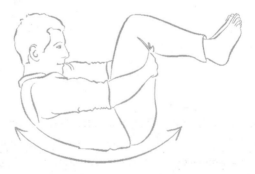

- Lie on a rug or a towel, lift your knees towards your chest, lift your head off the mat, and clasp your hands around your thighs. Rock forwards and back five or six times. Unclasp your hands and rest, then repeat.

Hip roll
- Lie on a rug or towel and stretch your arms out to either side. Lift your knees to your chest. Now, keeping your right shoulder touching the floor, lower your knees to the left, touching the floor if you can. Still keeping your right shoulder touching the floor, raise your knees to your chest, then lower them to the right, keeping your left shoulder on the floor. Repeat three times on each side.

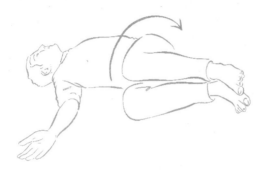

Loosen your shoulders
- Stand with your feet shoulder-width apart and move your shoulders around: up, down, round, forwards, and back – for about one minute.

Circulation-boosters
- Now get into practice for exercising in-flight. Turn to pages 92–3 and work through the four circulation-boosting exercises.

Thinking ahead

Preparing for a flight is essential. You need to assess your particular physical problems and requirements, and work out what you need to do and take. One person gets headaches, another has back problems. Everyone, men and women, however young and fit, needs to think ahead about ways of keeping the blood moving so that blood clots have no chance to form. An airline can only handle illness if it is alerted to a passenger's needs and can make the necessary preparation, so everyone should check the 'Fit to Fly?' list on pages 189–192 before booking a ticket.

Fear of flying is more common than we like to admit: it seems that 25 per cent of us suffer from some degree of nervousness. It is beyond the scope of this small book to tackle such a large problem, but the airlines can put you in touch with therapists who offer counselling and courses to help people deal with this phobia. However, considering the health risks of flying and taking steps to prevent illness may help nervous passengers to feel that they are taking realistic and positive action on their own behalf to deal with problems that more complacent passengers may fail to consider. What those passengers are doing is delegating all responsibility for their health to the airlines. The airlines, on the other hand, make safety their priority – with huge success. Every year 1,200 scheduled airlines fly 1.5 billion passengers to their destinations with scarcely an incident. The roads and railways do not approach their safety record.

CHAPTER TWO

Economy Class Syndrome and How to Prevent It

'Economy class syndrome' is the health issue the air traveller hears most about. It is an illness in which blood clots form in the veins of the legs – doctors call it deep-vein thrombosis, or 'DVT' for short. It is in the news because it *is* news, for although thrombosis is not a newly discovered illness, airlines and the medical profession have been slow to acknowledge a link between DVT and air travel. The travelling public began to hear about it only during the 1990s, when a huge expansion in the numbers of people flying long-haul resulted in an increase in the number of people being treated in hospitals serving international airports, and reports of sudden deaths made headlines. Travel-related DVT is a newly recognized type of thrombosis, so there no body of coordinated information and statistics on which physicians can draw. And because it is new, reports and articles about it in magazines and newspapers are contradictory and exaggerated. They raise more questions than they answer.

Travel-related DVT is a real medical condition, not an illness made up by the press. It deserves your serious attention because it can start off a sequence of events that can lead to death. Medical services at Heathrow, London's largest airport, report a serious emergency case of DVT approximately once a month, and you need to take action to prevent it from happening to you. On the other hand, the medical facilities of the world's airports are not clogged to a standstill with DVT victims on trolleys. It is vital to take evasive action, but also to be aware that many people fly without developing DVT, and a large number of people who develop symptoms while flying seem to recover quickly afterwards. What is certain is that this illness is most likely to affect certain categories of people. This chapter explores what doctors currently know about travel-related DVT, who is at risk, and what you can do to prevent it.

What is DVT?

Deep-vein thrombosis is the formation of a blood clot in a vein deep in the body. Thrombi, or blood clots, can form in the veins of the arms, the pelvis, and other parts of the body, but they form more commonly in the legs. A blood clot is not a danger in itself, but once it forms, it can grow so big that it blocks the flow of blood along the vein. Part of the blood clot can also be dislodged and carried in the blood to major organs, such as the lungs or even the brain. If it is large enough it may block a main artery in the lungs. This is a pulmonary embolism, and it is usually fatal.

It is important to record that as this book goes to press there is still no scientific proof of a link between air travel and DVT, the evidence is all circumstantial: the numbers of people flying long-haul increased substantially during the 1980s and 1990s, doctors have noticed a suspiciously large increase in the numbers of airline passengers showing symptoms of DVT.

Why 'economy class syndrome?'

British physicians recorded the occurrence of blood clots in the deep veins of the legs of people who slept in deck chairs while sheltering from night-time bombing in the early 1940s. Thorough investigation by television journalists working for the British television programme *Panorama* in 2001 turned up reports by physicians as early as the 1950s - when the first long-range passenger jets went into service. They interviewed a number of physicians in several different countries who had asked airlines to cooperate in research into the occurrence of the condition, but without success. The condition got scarcely a mention in textbooks on aviation medicine published before the 1990s. Only now is serious research being carried out.

A report produced in November 2000 by a UK Government committee tracked down the first appearance of the term 'economy class syndrome' to a paper published in a medical journal in 1977. Its two authors were reporting on cases of blood clots reaching the lungs of patients who had recently travelled economy class on international flights. The name they used has stuck, perhaps because many more people travel in economy class than in business or first class, so there are proportionally more recorded cases of DVT among economy-class passengers. Doctors believe that the cramped seating in economy class encourages the formation of blood clots in the leg veins of passengers flying for four hours or longer.

Do passengers travelling first class get DVT?

'Economy class syndrome' is a misleading term because people travelling long-distance in any type of transport or seat can suffer from DVT. In the USA it is still often called 'Dan Quayle syndrome' since the former US Vice-President, a frequent first-class flier, developed deep-vein thrombosis after a flight in 1994. In this book we have frequently called it 'travel-related DVT' or 'traveller's DVT'.

A study carried out in late 2000 in Norway suggests that people may develop travel-related DVT shortly after aircraft flying long-haul reach cruising height and the cabin becomes pressurized. Short-haul flights take so long to reach and descend from cruising height that they may spend considerably less than one hour at altitude and fully pressurized. More research is needed, however, before pressurization can be identified as a cause of this illness.

Can anyone get it?

It is estimated that one person in 10,000 under the age of sixty-five and one person in 1,000 over sixty-five will develop DVT whether or not they fly, because some people have a predisposition – they are more likely than others to develop blood clots in the veins. A major factor that puts you in the at-risk group for travel-related DVT is whether you or anyone in your family has had it in the past. Up to 20 per cent of people have minor abnormalities in the way their blood clots, and these people are believed to be more likely to get travel-related DVT in conditions that encourage it to develop. Records show that women are more likely to develop it than men, but a study carried out in London in 2000 found that almost as many men as women developed blood clots in the leg veins after a long-haul return flight. The study tested eighty-nine men and 142 women, all over fifty, none of whom had a history of blood clots; five men and seven women developed blood clots in the calf veins. Some doctors believe smokers are at a greater risk of travel-related DVT than non-smokers.

Who is most at risk?

Below is a full summary of people known to be at risk from developing travel-related DVT. If you are unsure of your risk category, check with your doctor, especially if you seem to fall into the medium- or high-risk groups. You can ask for a blood test to check for genetic factors that predispose people to develop DVT. If you are reading this as you travel, *don't panic*. Take sensible precautions (see below under **Can travel-related DVT be prevented?**) and check with a physician when you get back home.

More research needs to be carried out before doctors can make an accurate assessment of how many people are at risk. All they can do until then is make an educated guess. Guesses on record suggest that between one in ten and one in twenty air travellers flying long-haul are likely to develop travel-related DVT. In fact, flights of four hours or more put us at risk. The odds are on the low side if you fly long-haul for an occasional holiday and very much on the high side if you are a frequent medium- to long-haul flier.

Low risk:

- The over-forties: the likelihood of developing travel-related DVT increases with age.
- Very short, very tall, and obese travellers.
- Anyone who has experienced leg-swelling for any reason.
- People with recent minor leg injuries or who have recently had minor surgery to the body.
- Anyone who has recently been ill in bed or otherwise immobile for more than twenty-four hours.
- People with severe varicose veins.

Medium risk:

- Anyone who has recently developed heart disease or who has vascular disorders (problems affecting the blood vessels or the circulation).
- Women who are pregnant or taking the contraceptive pill, hormone replacement therapy (HRT), or oestrogen therapy for other reasons.
- Anyone who has recently had major leg surgery or suffered a major leg injury.
- Members of families with a history of DVT.

High risk:

- Anyone who has, or has previously experienced, DVT.
- People with a known tendency towards increased blood clotting or other blood-clotting abnormalities.
- Patients who have recently had major body surgery or a serious injury to the body.
- Stroke victims.
- Cancer patients and anyone who has been treated for cancer.
- Anyone who cannot move either or both legs.

Can travel-related DVT be prevented?

You can take many actions to prevent travel-related DVT from developing if you are in the no-risk or low–medium-risk categories. Below is a summary of preventive measures, and they are explained in more detail in the following pages. In addition, many of the measures to prevent back pain (see Chapter 3) also help prevent travel-related DVT, and many of the exercises in Chapter 4 boost circulation in the legs and feet to prevent blood clots from forming.

It is important to be sure of your degree of risk. Travellers at medium risk should check with a physician regarding precautions to take before travelling. It may not be possible to prevent the development of travel-related DVT in high-risk people. You must consult a physician before travelling and be prepared to postpone the flight or use a different method of transport. Your doctor may pronounce you fit to fly if you have an injection of low molecular weight heparin (a natural substance which breaks down blood clots) before flying, and take all the precautions listed for lower-risk categories above. However, it is essential to report your condition to the airline when booking your ticket so that cabin crew can be aware of possible needs.

- Drink plenty of still water during the flight. Dehydration thickens the blood and this may encourage blood clots to form.
- Do not drink alcohol or many drinks containing caffeine, before or during the flight.
- Do not smoke immediately before or after the flight, or during the flight if smoking is permitted, or while on a stopover.
- Wear special compression socks during the flight (see page 42).
- If you are tall, sit in an aisle seat and stretch your legs into the aisle frequently during the flight.
- If the edge of the seat is not rounded, has a raised edge, and cuts into the backs of your legs, find something to rest your feet on so you can lift your knees clear of the cushion, or pad the edge of the cushion with something soft.
- Do not sit still for long: move around in your seat and get up and walk when you can.
- Do the key circulation-booster exercises on pages 92–4 at least once an hour during the flight.
- If you want to sleep, follow the instructions on pages 78–80, and sleep for short periods only if you are not lying flat. Do not take sleeping pills.

- Taking a 75 mg aspirin an hour or two before you fly, unless you suffer from stomach ulcers or from stomach irritations such as indigestion, or you are allergic to aspirin, is widely recommended by physicians specializing in aviation medicine. However, check with your doctor before you fly.

Compression socks

Do not wear knee-high socks or holdup stockings with an elastic top that grips the leg above or below the knee. They impede circulation and encourage blood clots to develop. Aviation medicine physicians recommend that passengers buy special compression socks to wear in-flight. These were designed by vascular surgeons (who specialize in disorders of the blood vessels) for their patients to wear after surgery. The socks grip the leg, but the grip is strongest at the ankle and lessens gradually towards the top. This compresses the leg veins, forcing the blood up to the heart. Compression socks are not the same as the support stockings women wear to prevent or alleviate varicose veins. Support stockings do not grip strongly enough in the lower part of the leg to be effective in preventing blood clots from forming.

The research into travel-related DVT carried out in London in 2000 by John Scurr, a vascular surgeon, gave compression socks to one group of air passengers to wear on long-haul flights. None developed blood clots in the leg veins. These findings do not prove the efficacy of compression socks, however. To be accepted as valid proof, the experiment must be repeated elsewhere and the findings compared. Nevertheless, vascular surgeons believe that compression socks help prevent blood clots from forming, and recommend them for flights of more than four hours.

Compression socks sound as if they look awful, but they are made of light, modern elasticated yarn and come in black and flesh colour. They are available on prescription from primary care doctors and practice nurses, and are sold (in standard sizes) by pharmacists and surgical suppliers, in department stores and at airport and airline shops. Put them on just before or after boarding the aircraft and take them off when you reach your destination. Buy some to wear if your job involves standing for long periods and you will be less likely to develop varicose veins – thought to be a risk factor for travel-related DVT.

TRAVEL-RELATED DVT: THE STORY SO FAR

DVT marks one of the frontiers of medicine, because physiologists have not yet discovered why blood clots sometimes form in an otherwise healthy vein. Clotting is a normal, healthy process: the blood clots to stop the body from bleeding to death after a cut. But a blood clot (called a thrombus) sometimes forms in a vein or an artery with no apparent damage.

The role of the veins

The heart pumps blood along the network of arteries to every part of the body. On its way around the body, the blood passes through the lungs, where it absorbs oxygen, then flows along branching networks of smaller and smaller blood vessels to nourish the organs and tissues.

The veins collect deoxygenated blood from the tissues and return it to the heart. In the tissues, the deoxygenated blood is channelled into tiny blood vessels and carried, along with wastes released by the cells, into networks of progressively larger blood vessels. These transport it to nearby veins, which carry it back to the heart and lungs to be relieved of its wastes, resupplied with oxygen, and recirculated.

If thrombi, or blood clots, occur in the micro-vessels serving the body tissues, they usually cause little damage. But when they form in a vein or an artery they can cause serious blockages. Once blood clots form, they grow, because particles tend to stick to them, and some grow large enough to block the flow of blood through the blood vessel. Large fragments can break off and be carried in the blood flow to the lungs, the heart, or the brain, where they may block the circulation and inhibit breathing or cause a stroke.

Why blood clots develop in the leg veins

The heart pumps blood along the arteries under great pressure, but that pressure lessens as the blood reaches the tissues, and by the time it makes its return journey along the veins the pressure is much lower. Blood from the feet has to travel all the way up the legs and through the abdomen to the heart against the force of gravity – worse than cycling up Mount Kilimanjaro from a climbing start.

To help it on its climb up from the feet, the deeper veins of the legs are lined with valves, which allow the blood to flow upwards, then open out to prevent the flow from reversing downwards. These valves have a tough job, especially if their owner has to stand all day at work, and they can become enlarged, twisted, or distorted. These are called varicose veins. Blood clots often start in stagnant blood around defective veins.

Even if you have healthy veins, your ankles swell and your feet feel tight in your shoes at the end of a day on your feet – or sitting in an aircraft seat – without walking about much. If you stand or sit still for a long time, the flow of blood from feet to heart slows. The veins in your legs and feet widen, acting as a reservoir for blood that is stagnating or pooling there because there is no pressure behind it to push it back up to the heart.

Muscle power prevents blood clots

To stay healthy, blood needs to keep moving. In recent years physicians have understood that lounging around in bed – even for a very good reason such as a major operation or giving birth to triplets – needs to be discouraged, because slow blood flow gives blood clots time to form in the deep veins of the legs. No sooner have you come round from your anaesthetic or sunk into a welcome postpartum sleep, than nurses haul you out of bed and make you walk briskly around to restore tone to your veins and get your blood circulation back to speed to prevent blood clots forming.

Muscle power is the body's natural mechanism for preventing blood clots from developing. The deep veins of the legs lie between two muscle groups, one close to the surface and one deep inside the calf. As you walk, these muscles contract and relax, and as they do so they press against the veins, compressing and releasing, acting as a pump to move the blood up the vein to the heart.

Walking is intensely beneficial. It speeds up the return of blood from feet to heart, preventing distension of the veins and pooling of the blood. This increases the output of blood from the heart, improving blood flow to the brain and to the hands and feet. It keeps you warmer, gives the brain the oxygen it needs to function efficiently, and nourishes the body cells more completely.

Exercise also makes you more resistant to disease. It stimulates the body's second major circulatory system, called the lymphatic system. Lymph is a colourless fluid that circulates around the whole body, carrying nourishment to all the tissues and taking wastes away, and it also carries lymphocytes – cells that fight disease and infection all around the body. Inactivity also slows the circulation of lymph.

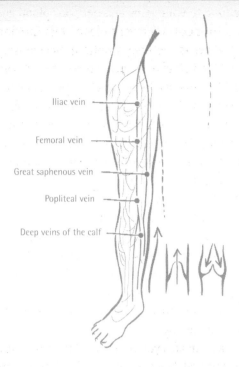

Iliac vein

Femoral vein

Great saphenous vein

Popliteal vein

Deep veins of the calf

There are veins at different levels in the legs – the longest vein in the body is the great saphenous vein, which runs from the groin down to the feet. This vein is fairly close to the surface, and although clots can form inside it, thrombi in superficial veins tend to stick to the walls, so fragments rarely break off and move into the lungs. Blood clots that form in the smaller veins deep in the legs, especially those in the calves, are more worrying, since blood is more likely to stagnate in this network, and blood clots may form which may travel to the lungs.

Exercising in-flight

The idea of exercising while sitting in an aircraft seat was inconceivable only a year or two ago, but now that the danger of travel-related DVT is understood, everyone concerned with airline health is looking for ways to make it possible. Exercising in economy class is especially problematical. If you are tall, you can't move your legs. You are wary of kicking your neighbour. If you are short, your feet don't reach the floor.

Yet when it comes to stimulating circulation in the legs and feet, simple exercises involving small movements are surprisingly effective if you do them once every half hour to an hour. Pushing the feet hard down against the floor, lifting the toes, rotating the ankles, are all movements that get the blood circulating. These movements are major components of the key circulation-boosting exercises which begin the programme of exercises in Chapter 4. Try out these exercises and you will find they relieve the stiffness that comes from sitting still, and they will make you feel more comfortable. You should also be able to walk up and down the aisle of the aircraft now and again during a flight – but beware! Turbulence is an invisible air disturbance that high-flying aircraft sometimes run into. The aircraft is designed to ride it out, but passengers in the cabin can get jolted as if they were riding a bucking bronco. Always hold hard on to seats as you walk down an aircraft aisle.

As this book goes to press, innovation in the area of

in-flight exercise is beginning to hit the headlines. The Airogym is a small rubber exercise mat which gives resistance when you press down, making your legs and feet work harder as you exercise. It was designed by a British Airways pilot after one of his passengers was taken ill with travel-related DVT. Vascular surgeons confirm that it can increase blood flow through the deep leg veins by as much as 50 per cent. The Back Shop's Stepfit is a similar device which has small plastic spikes built in to massage your feet as you exercise. Massage techniques are included in Chapter 4, but massage is always deeper and more effective if you use a massage stick. All these devices cost very little.

Exercise mats could be a boon to teenagers, elderly people, and anyone else whose legs are short and whose feet do not reach the floor. Sitting with the backs of the legs pressing down against the edge of the seat compresses major veins and arteries at the back of the knees, and this can stop the blood flow and encourage travel-related DVT. This is why short stature is one of the at-risk categories for travel-related DVT. A lightweight exercise mat like the Airogym and the Stepfit could provide a raised level on which you can rest your feet and lift your knees above the seat edge.

How do you recognize travel-related DVT?

Blood clots may develop while you are in the air, but also – it is important to remember – from two to four

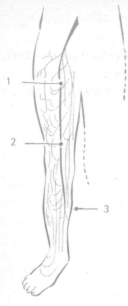

weeks after a flight. If you are a frequent flier you should check regularly for signs. Just to confuse everyone, doctors included, blood clots in the calf, where the deep veins lie between two sets of muscles, often produce no symptoms at all and it can be difficult to tell whether anything is wrong. Check each area of both legs in turn, looking carefully at the skin surface in a good light, and check the back of your thighs in a mirror. Are there any areas of redness? Any swelling? Can you feel any pains or cramps? If you are a bit squeamish, skip the detailed list of symptoms that follows. But remember where it is and come back to it if you have any strange symptoms in your legs.

The upper thighs

A clot in the iliac veins (1) affects the blood supply to the whole leg, so produces obvious symptoms. Check for:

- A hard cordlike area in your groin and in the centre of the back of your thigh.
- Swelling; a feeling of warmth in the swollen area.
- Red discoloration on the skin surface of the thigh.
- Severe pain affecting the whole leg.

The thighs just above the knees

A clot in the femoral vein (2) will affect the whole of your leg below it. Check for:

- A hard, cordlike structure at the back of your knee.
- Swelling; warmth or heat in the swollen area.
- Red discoloration on the skin anywhere from the knee downwards.
- Pain from the knee down.

The calves

A clot in the deep veins of the calves (3) often produces severe and persistent swelling of the ankles. Even if you have no symptoms, however, you should still check for a clot by seeing whether you have the following symptoms and doing the test:

- Swelling or tenderness when you feel your calves from just below the knee down to your ankle.
- Pain when you stand or walk.
- Test: hold on to a bathroom rail or a chair back and lift your left leg, keeping it straight, and dorsiflexing your foot (bending it towards you). Repeat the test, this time lifting your leg with the knee bent. Then test your right leg in the same way. Pain in your leg when you keep your leg straight, but not when you bend it, could be a sign of travel-related DVT.

The chest

It is possible for a blood clot to reach the lung or other part of the body without any preceding signs of travel-related DVT. Just to be extra-safe, be aware of any of the following signs. If they occur, go straight to a hospital emergency department, explain that you have been on a long-haul flight, and describe your symptoms:

- Unfamiliar sensations in the chest (sometimes described as a kind of internal tugging or pulling feeling) accompanied by pain.
- Pain in the chest which is severe or worsens steadily.
- Unfamiliar and worsening breathlessness.
- Coughing up blood.

When to ask for help

Don't panic if you think you have symptoms. All the signs of travel-related DVT are also symptoms of other conditions, some of them very straightforward. The ankles often swell when you sit still for a long time, and the swelling subsides when you walk around for a while. Pain may be due to muscle cramp, also brought on by prolonged sitting, or something equally simple. Swelling, pain, and other symptoms in both legs are much less likely to be a sign of DVT than if one leg only is affected. But you need to be sure.

■ **If you develop symptoms in-flight**, alert a flight attendant. Judging by reports from people we have interviewed, this may produce nothing more than polite concern. However, more and more airlines are training their cabin crews in how to deal with travel-related DVT, so that if you are flying with one of the large international airlines, you will almost certainly receive more informed treatment. Here are a few things you can do if you develop symptoms in-flight:

● Get up and walk around if you can.
● Drink plenty of still water during the remainder of the flight.
● **Do not** take an aspirin. (It is important not to take aspirin if you develop symptoms of travel-related DVT. Your condition may have to be treated with different medication and aspirin could interfere with its effects.)
● If you are wearing knee-high socks, take them off. If you have or can obtain from the flight attendants a compression sock, put it on the affected leg.
● Ask to be moved to a first-class seat. If none is available, ask to sit in an aisle seat and stretch your legs into the aisle.
● Do the key circulation-boosting leg exercises shown on pages 92–4.
● Stay awake for the rest of the flight, unless you can lie full-length with your leg raised 15 centimetres (6 inches) above your head. It is very important not to fall asleep in a cramped sitting position.
● When you arrive at your destination, ask the flight attendants or airport staff to put you in touch with the airport medical services.

■ **If you notice symptoms while at the airport**, ask for the airport medical facilities. You may be taken to see a physician, or you may be taken to the nearest hospital accident and emergency department. If you are in a foreign country you may need to pay or have medical insurance (see appendix, pages 192–3).

■ **If you notice symptoms at home, after your trip,** contact your doctor at once by telephone or by visiting the surgery, or go straight to a hospital accident and emergency department. You must remember to tell the hospital staff you have travelled by air recently.

How is DVT treated?

Whether you are seen at an airport medical facility or a nearby hospital, or you see a physician at home, treatment will be very similar. Blood clots in the veins are not always fatal, but they can have serious consequences if they are not treated immediately and correctly. This is what generally happens:

- The physician will examine your leg, checking for areas of hardness, redness, swelling and pain, ask whether you or anyone in your family has had blood-clotting disorders, and how your symptoms developed.
- Remember to say if you have taken medication for travel sickness, heparin, aspirin, or sleeping tablets, what dosage, and roughly when. If you are examined abroad by a physician who does not speak your language, write down the name of the medication or, if you can, show the medication or its packaging.
- If your leg is painful, the doctor will give you an analgesic that does not contain aspirin.
- You will normally have an ultrasound scan so the blood clot can be examined. An ultrasound scan uses

sound waves to produce an image of the veins inside the body. It is completely safe and you cannot feel the scan – it causes no pain at all. A range of other tests, such as venography (any blood clots show up when a coloured dye is passed into a vein) may be carried out if ultrasound is not available.

- When the doctor has assessed your veins you will be given an anticoagulant injection (anticoagulants are drugs that dissolve blood clots).
- You will be hospitalized for close monitoring and treatment. You rest in bed with your leg raized 15 centimetres (6 inches) above your head, and you are given painkillers and anticoagulant injections. You will be in hospital for five or six days, but if there are complications, you may need to stay for longer.

How long does the treatment last?

After the emergency is over you will need to continue treatment with anticoagulants. Its duration will depend on your illness, but it may last for three months or more. Anyone who normally attends an alternative therapy clinic may well find that travel-related DVT is too new for alternative practitioners to have tried and tested treatments to offer, and reputable therapists will advise you to see an orthodox physician. Acupuncture and therapeutic massage can help you while you are under medical treatment, and these therapies are quite safe. The gentle exercise systems, such as daiji (t'ai chi), yoga, and pilates body-conditioning will help your circulation. Be sure to tell your teacher about your travel-related DVT because you may need to avoid strenuous movements. Make gentle leg exercises part of your daily routine for life and you may never have another travel-related DVT episode.

- When you leave hospital you will need to attend a weekly clinic to continue anticoagulant treatment.
- A physiotherapist may give you leg and foot exercises to improve blood flow and to strengthen the muscles of your legs and feet.

Does DVT recur?

DVT is a worrying illness, but do bear in mind that many thousands of people are thought to develop the condition in different circumstances without suspecting that they have it. The blood clots that form may be tiny and they may break down naturally, leaving no trace. If more serious clots are diagnosed but not treated properly, they can damage veins, and that can encourage new clots to form. In extreme cases, DVT can cause permanent damage, so that the affected leg develops permanent swelling and painful ulcers, and walking becomes difficult.

Once you have experienced DVT, the risk of another episode is always present. And that means the risk of an embolism or travelling blood clot fragment lodging in the lung or another organ. Write your name in your mind's eye on the at-risk list, and always take precautions. Good, brisk leg exercise must become a daily routine: make a point of walking instead of driving, and climb stairs instead of taking the lift. Start regular gentle exercise or sport. These activities will benefit your whole life, and as a bonus they will keep you mobile into old age. Consult your physician if you are ever in doubt. And in addition:

DOs and DON'Ts
- Never sit with your knees or ankles crossed.
- Do not sit in deck chairs and avoid chairs that cut into your legs just above the knee.
- If you have to stand in a queue for a long time, move your weight from one leg to the other, and exercise your feet while you stand, raising the toes and then the heels, pressing your toes into the ground and then releasing them.
- Wear compression socks whenever you think you may need to sit still for a long period – in a film or a lecture, at a play or a concert.
- Eat a healthy diet to maintain a healthy body/mass index.
- If you are a smoker, stop smoking permanently.
- Check with a physician specializing in aviation medicine if you contemplate a long-haul flight in the future. If you are given the go-ahead, check different airlines and choose the one offering the widest seat pitch. Think of flying business class, if you can. In-flight, follow the advice in Chapter 3 on caring for your back, as well as all the advice in this chapter on avoiding travel-related DVT.

Support Organizations

As this book goes to press news has surfaced of action being brought against airlines by a legal firm in Sydney, Australia, who report that they have had enquiries from more than 2,500 victims of travel-related DVT. At the same time, support organizations for victims of travel-related DVT and their relatives are being set up in many countries. For up-to-date information about action and support, contact the Aviation Health Institute (AHI), listed on page 196.

CHAPTER THREE
Back Stress, Strain, Sprain and Pain

'Your back kills you' was one frequent flier's worst memory of travelling long-haul in economy class, before she upgraded. Back pain is ordinary, and people just ignore it like they put up with colds and flu. But they don't realize how much strain flying puts on the lower back and how much damage that can do. Back trouble is an occupational hazard for pilots, who know that if they ignore the twinges, these may eventually cause serious damage, disability, loss of mobility, and suspension of the medical certificate they need to fly. If your back is weak, if you sometimes get back pain, if you are a frequent flier and if you fly long-haul in economy class, flying can damage your spine. If you are reading this crammed into an undersized cabin seat with your destination several hours away, you need to take action to protect your back. This chapter explains the problem and focuses on things you can do to keep your back comfortable in-flight.

The airborne skeleton

Back pain is one of the conditions doctors see most often in their surgeries. It is the leading disability of people in Western industrial countries, so much so that some experts are now calling it an epidemic. In the USA it is the No.1 problem for under-45s, and the UK has more than 15 million sufferers – almost 25 per cent of the population. So no wonder backache is the physical complaint most often reported to airlines.

Yet flying is hard on the back even if you do not

have a back problem. Why? The short answer is that the body is not built to sit for hours without moving. Watch people in a room and they move a lot, sitting and standing, walking, bending and turning. Tribal peoples squat, kneel, and sit on the ground. All these movements stretch and strengthen the spine. Keep moving to keep your back pain-free.

Sitting may feel more comfortable than standing, but in the long run it is extra work for the body. When you stand naturally, the weight of your upper body is transmitted by the lumbar vertebrae (the large bones of your lower spine) around your pelvis to your leg joints, then down your legs to your feet and into the ground. But when you sit down, your pelvis rotates backwards, and the weight of your upper body is borne by your lumbar spine. This puts immense strain on the discs of cartilage that separate the lumbar vertebrae, on the ligaments that tie them together, and on the muscles that hold them upright. Looked at from the lumbar spine's point of view, it is hardly surprising that after putting up with all this extra stress for an hour or two, it raises hell. Aching is the back's way of complaining.

Adding to this discomfort is pressure from the seat you are sitting on. Airline seats and backs are padded with foam. When you sit still for a long time the foam gradually compresses, pushing out all the air, so that eventually you feel as if you are sitting on rock. Aircraft seat designers call this process 'seepage'.

Economy-class seats are usually narrow, and shallow

from back to front, so that you cannot move around easily when sitting in one, especially if you are tall or large. Seepage makes hollows in the foam where your body presses against it, and those hollows hold you still more firmly in place. Seats in business and first class, on the other hand, are wide and deep enough to give plenty of squirming room. Squirming is healthy because it encourages the circulation of fluids around the spinal cord and the brain. The cerebrospinal fluid cushions the brain and spinal cord from jarring as you move. As it circulates it carries sodium, chloride, potassium, calcium and other nutrients from the central areas of the brain to the brain stem at its base, around the spinal cord, and out to the veins on the brain's surface.

To fly long-haul is to subject your back to these extreme conditions for an abnormally long time. Back pain is usually a sign of back strain, so even if your back is strong and flexible, very frequent flying could perhaps be the start of a back condition that will show up in future years. And if you are one of the large percentage of people who already have a back problem, sitting abnormally still in a restricting cabin seat for eight hours or more may be making an existing problem worse. A distinguished physician who works with pilots reported recently in a professional magazine that many pilots endure back pain for years and see a doctor only when the pain is unendurable. By that time the damage is so bad, they often need surgery.

Many people occasionally have an acute attack of back pain because they wrench a ligament, a muscle or a tendon playing football, moving furniture – or perhaps from twisting round awkwardly to pick up a heavy suitcase from the floor just behind them. Twenty-four hours lying on a firm mattress with knees bent up, plus medication and a week or two of massage and physio-therapy usually cures the problem, but you have to take care not to let the same thing happen again or it may become chronic.

The kind of back pain you notice after a long air trip may have been developing for years. It almost always results from habitual poor posture: sitting at badly designed work stations, slumping in front of the TV, walking with head poked forwards and shoulders hunched. If you like to play tennis, swim, or work out, you strengthen the muscles that hold your spine upright, so the odd hour spent slumped in front of a computer game, upper body all bunched up, will not do lasting damage. But if you hate to exercise, you let the muscles, tendons and ligaments that hold the bones of your spine in place weaken. Poor posture plus weak spinal muscles adds up to a back injury waiting to happen.

Basic spinal maintenance:
Keep your back strong with good posture and regular exercise. If your back is flexible it will withstand the stresses and strains of a long-haul flight with minimal damage.

- Check the physical condition of your back: get it checked by a doctor, a physiotherapist, a chiropractor, or a therapist specializing in Alexander technique or pilates.
- Correct any weakness by doing strengthening exercises regularly, supervised by a physiotherapist or a teacher of pilates, Alexander technique, or yoga.
- Keep your back strong through regular exercise or sport. Swimming (crawl or back stroke but not breast stroke) is good exercise for the spine if you are pregnant or in your later years and unused to exercise.

Lifting and lowering luggage

Do your shoulders and back feel sore after hauling your luggage to the airport? How do you pick up heavy bags? Do you stagger to the car or bus with one in each hand, another hung over your shoulder? What part of your body do you use to lift them up into a rack? What is your body posture when you put them down on the floor? Back strain (damage to muscles and the tendons that attach them to bones) and sprains (damage to joints between bones and the ligaments that hold them in place) may also result from lifting and dropping heavy loads using what physiotherapists call 'improper back mechanics'. If you bend forwards to pick up a heavy bag, keeping your legs straight as you lift it, you put a tremendous load on your lumbar spine.

Train yourself to be more aware of the mechanics of your spine:

● Keep your back straight when lifting a packed bag: bend your knees, grasp the object, and lift or lower it by straightening your knees. Your calf and thigh muscles do the work, not your back, so the load is transmitted down your legs to your feet and into the ground. Hold the bag close to your body as you lift, and raise it only up to your chest – lifting heavy loads to shoulder height can stress your upper spine. Ask someone to help you lift it into an overhead locker. And do not lift and twist round while holding the bag: if you have to put it down to one side, keep holding it close to your chest, turn your whole body left or right, then lower it bending your knees.

MUSCLE SPASM

If you have painful twinges in your spine now or when you disembark, they are probably caused by muscle spasm. In time, if they are not corrected, slouching, poor back mechanics, weak back structures, and recurrent injury can cause permanent pain and irreparable damage. The spinal cord is made up of major nerves running from the brain through the middle of the spine and out through openings in the vertebrae to all parts of the body. The brain responds quickly to signals that seem to report discomfort from any of the spinal nerves and one of its reactions is to send muscles in the affected area into painful spasm to try to limit the damage they seem to be doing.

■ **Relax your back muscles,** because the spine and brain are so closely linked, period pains and gynaecological problems in women, prostate trouble in men, tiredness, tension, and emotional problems can all spark off backache. If your back is killing you when you get to your destination, try these remedies:

- Body massage relaxes the major muscle groups of the body, restoring normal circulation to the muscles of the spine by releasing tension and reducing spasm.
- Heat treatment, from a warm bath to infrared treatment, will often soothe muscle spasms.
- If the twinges continue or worsen, see a doctor. You may need strong painkillers and antispasmodic drugs or muscle relaxants.

SLIPPED DISK

If you experience excruciating pain in your lower back, it may be caused by a slipped disk. This is usually the result of misuse of the spine over a long period and is not caused by air travel, but the strain of prolonged sitting in cramped conditions can cause the disk to press on a major nerve, and this is what causes the agonizing pain. The disks are cushions of cartilage which separate pairs of vertebrae (spinal bones) and act as shock absorbers as you move about. They have a soft, springy centre surrounded by a tough outer covering. Poor posture and jarring movements may cause a disk to move out of place, then the outer membrane

may be punctured by normal movement of the surrounding bones. When this happens the soft centre
may be squeezed through the outer membrane and
press on nerves. Fragments of the disk may break off,
irritating nearby nerves. If the nerves become pinched
or damaged they may stop communicating properly
with other parts of the body. If the legs and feet are
affected, mobility is impaired. Surgery may be the only
way of correcting these serious conditions, relieving
the pain and restoring normal mobility.

Signs of injury:
Back injury may seem to occur suddenly for no reason.
It may have been building up for a long time and have
worsened suddenly after a period of stress. If you
experience any of these symptoms, see a doctor immediately. You may notice some of the symptoms after a
long-haul flight, but they may occur at any time. Seek
treatment immediately to prevent further damage.
These days, microsurgery can usually relieve the pain
and restore normal mobility.

- Occasional twinges somewhere in your back seem to
  have become more frequent and they often shoot
  off down your buttock or leg.
- Your lower back aches much more than it used to
  and the pain is more intense, so you have to lie
  down. The pain may be so bad it makes you sweat.
- You get bouts of back pain with numbness, tingling,
  or stiffness in your legs, feet, arms, or hands. Ask to
  see an orthopaedic specialist.

- You find you cannot straighten up after bending and the pain in your lower back is intense if you try to move. You need immediate hospital admission and an epidural injection to relieve the symptoms.

Uncommon back problems

A small percentage of people have deformities of the spine and some people develop degenerative bone diseases such as osteoarthritis. These can cause backache and long-distance air travel, especially in economy seats, may well cause severe pain. It is better not to travel by air in economy class: consider another form of transport, or travel in premium economy, if available, or business class. However, arthritis usually develops in later life, whereas backache is the most common medical condition of the under-45s, in whom such diseases are rare. Poor posture and weak back muscles will always make them worse.

- If you have osteoarthritis or any other medical condition affecting your spine, see your doctor before booking a long-haul trip to discuss the possible effects of such a trip on your back.

Are you sitting comfortably?

If you are sitting while reading this, perhaps in an aircraft seat, at home, or in your lunch-break at work, take a moment to think about how you are sitting, and how you got into that position. Did you drop on to the seat sideways and bend forwards with the book on your knee, back rounded and head bent? Or did you throw yourself half on to the seat without looking behind, then flop back, curving your back into

Slumping and slouching load as much strain on to your lumbar spine as sitting immobile in a cramped economy-class seat on a long-haul flight – but they do it much more cheaply.

the chair back and holding the book up? If you stay in that position, how will your body feel in half an hour?

If you are sitting upright with your shoulders pressing back towards the chair back, head lifting from the crown, you will still feel comfortable in half an hour. Your sitting posture enables your body to balance the weight of its upper half and transmit it downwards in the most energy-efficient way, without overloading your lower spine.

Balanced sitting is not sitting up with the back ramrod straight, a book balancing on the head, as young ladies were taught at nineteenth-century academies. In its natural position, standing or sitting, the spine has three curves, an inward or forward curve in the lumbar area, an outward or backward curve in the upper back, and a shallow curve forwards at the neck. These curves distribute your upper body weight evenly down to the chair, and they contribute to the spine's marvellous flexibility.

The curves are formed by the upper twenty-four of the spine's thirty-three bones or vertebrae, from the atlas and axis, which support and move the skull, to

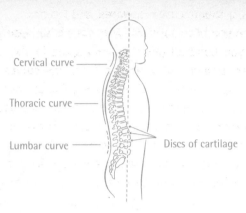

Cervical curve

Thoracic curve

Lumbar curve

Discs of cartilage

the bottommost of the five lumbar vertebrae, which joins the back of the pelvis. They are separated by cartilage disks and tied together in pairs and threes by ligaments. The cartilage allows each pair of vertebrae to bend just a little way back and forwards, left and right. These tiny movements enable the separate bones to work together, each contributing its quota of movement to enable the spine to bend back and to either

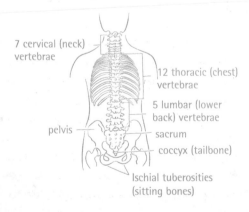

7 cervical (neck) vertebrae

12 thoracic (chest) vertebrae

5 lumbar (lower back) vertebrae

pelvis

sacrum

coccyx (tailbone)

Ischial tuberosities (sitting bones)

side, twist round, curve forwards, and lift up.

When you bend forwards with your elbows on your knees, you bend all joints in your spine in the same direction, ironing out your spine's natural curves. The same happens when you mould your body into the chair back. Your middle spine presses hard against the chair back, your pelvis is rotated right back, and the vertebrae of your lumbar or lower spine have no support. The weight of your upper body cascades downwards, pressing your buttock muscles against the chair seat, pushing your thighs forwards. Seat designers call this pushing action 'shear', and you know when it is happening because it causes your clothes to ride up beneath your thighs. Your spine is immobilized, and its discomfort will soon make itself felt.

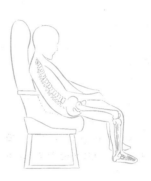

Are you sitting upright? Practise sitting up, right now, and you will be able to sit for far longer without discomfort. If you sit upright correctly, and then recline the seat, you will incline backwards from the sitting bones and this will not load extra weight on to your lumbar spine.

● Sit with the sacrum – the bone at the base of the spine – close up against the back of the chair and your head lifted from the crown. This allows your spine to assume its natural S-curves between the two and the weight of your upper body to fall on the sitting bones (their medical name is 'ischial tuberosities') at the base of your pelvis.

- When you sit upright, your trunk (your body from the hip bones to the neck) forms an angle of 90° to your thighs. The weight of your upper body is then transmitted along your spine, around your pelvis, and down to the sitting bones, to disperse into the seat.

- Your heels and toes rest on the floor, and your thighs lie parallel to the floor. Your legs and thighs are at right angles to each other. The angle between your thighs and your pelvis should be 90° to 100°; any greater and the weight of your upper body is thrown on to the lumbar spine instead of being transmitted down to the sitting bones.

- Your head needs to be support-ed upright by the headrest. Allowing it to tilt right back throws extra stress on to the cervical or neck vertebrae.

- Keep your sacrum up against the chair back when you adjust the chair into the recline posi-tion. You will then recline with it directly from the sitting bones instead of bending backwards from the hips.

How average are you?

Aircraft cabin seats are designed for a mythical 'average passenger', yet bodies have very different shapes and dimensions. Seats in first and business class have adjustable headrests, armrests, footrests and other appendages which enable them to change position to some degree to suit the different sizes and shapes of their occupants. Seats in economy class have scarcely any of these accommodating features. Depending on the airline and their age, these seats may be larger or smaller, wider or narrower, and better or less well cushioned, but the essentials (seat height and width, height and length of the armrests, and back support) will not be variable. Tall people suffer because if the armrests are too low they tend to twist their upper body sideways. Children, and people with short legs, may be uncomfortable if their feet do not reach the floor. Statistics show that the world population is increasing in size and weight – 25 per cent of Americans are clinically obese – so many people will find the seats too tight. Size and weight put great stress on the lower back, so larger passengers and women in the last trimester of pregnancy need to take all the care they can to support the lower back.

However upright your sitting posture, it is a depressing fact that, if you travel in economy class, you are likely to be uncomfortable if the dimensions of your body are different from those of the cabin seat. The biggest problem is often the chair back. To increase passenger comfort, aircraft seats often have padding, intended to support the back. The problem is that anyone who does not fit the average profile may find that the padding is uncomfortably positioned directly above or below the hollow in the lower back. Economy class seats often have minimal padding, and this is also uncomfortable.

Customize your seat

The answer to these discomforts is to think of the aircraft seat as raw sitting material which you need to customize to fit the needs of your own body. Some airlines give out pillows and these will be helpful if you are reading this while travelling. But it is sensible to work out in advance exactly what your body needs and to board the aircraft well equipped to supply those needs.

The first thing to worry about is your lumbar spine. When you sit, the backward tilt of your pelvis increases the inward or forward curve of your spine at the level of your lower back, and it makes the outward or backward curve higher up the spine more pronounced. If you sit for just a short time, this effect will cause no problems. Your spine is flexible and will adjust easily when you stand and move about. But if you sit for a long time, it will make your back ache. To prevent this, you need support – some padding – but to be effective it must be positioned in exactly the right place: it must support your spine from the point where it curves inwards, round about your waist, to the point where it starts to curve outwards, roughly level with your lower ribs. Its effect is to prevent your pelvis from tilting too far back and increasing the upper curve in your back. It is quite easy to feel with your hands the points where your spine starts to curve, but if you need to be sure, sit in a straight-back chair beside a long mirror and look at the shape your back makes when you lean against the chair.

The next stage is to experiment. Put a small cushion at the level of your lumbar curve and sit back against it. As you sit back, the curve deepens a little, a condition called 'lordosis'. Instinct will tell you whether you need to move the cushion or whether you need a fatter one. Trust your instinct: if you dislike lumbar support and you are comfortable without it, your back probably does not need it.

If you are sitting in an aircraft seat, ask for an airline pillow and do the same experiment. If the seat is padded, but the padding is in the wrong place for you, placing the pillow in the hollow of your lower back will make the seat more comfortable.

It is a good idea to do a little research before a long-haul flight. There are many aids for back problems to be found on the market. The larger surgical suppliers' stores often have a good range you can try out, and you can find suppliers' catalogues on the Internet. London

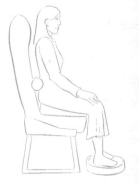

has the excellent Back Shop (details on page 195), which retails products from many different manufacturers. Staff will advise on support suitable for your individual back.

No one wants to board an aircraft loaded up with cushions. You need to look for something lightweight and small, perhaps inflatable, that will fit easily in your hand luggage until you need it. Aircraft regulations are very strict: anything you take on board in your hand luggage must be able to be stowed in a locker during take-off and landing. A lumbar roll is a simple cylinder of foam rubber designed to support the lower back. The Back Shop sells the SitFit, a versatile squashy round cushion 33 or 36 centimetres (13 or 14 inches) in diameter. It is designed to sit on, to raise the height of your pelvis slightly – which may make you more comfortable if you are sitting on a seat with inbuilt lumbar support in the wrong place for your back – and it redistributes your weight towards your knees. You can also use it as a lumbar support, and if you are short, you can put it on the floor and rest your feet on it.

When buying back care aids to lean against or to sit on, think about the materials they are made of. If your body is going to lean on a material for long stretches of time, the material must allow it to breathe. Materials that do this best have a pile, like velvet or sheepskin, which allows air to circulate through the fibres. Chair leather has grooves scored in it for the same purpose. Cotton and linen are absorbent, but smooth rubber and plastic will feel rather sweaty after a while. For this reason some back supports can be used just for half an hour or so at a time, unless they have an absorbent cover.

Dynamic sitting

You sit perfectly upright, your lower back well supported, for an hour or more. And then you feel uncomfortable. Your back aches. Why? An American Professor of Orthopaedics, Rowland G. Hazard, reports having studied this problem to try to help his patients. On a long journey he sat back against a cushion, well positioned against his lumbar spine, and felt very comfortable ... for a while. So he took the cushion away, and that made him feel comfortable again ... but only for a while.

The fact is that to keep your spine comfortable, you need to keep it in action. Moving about is the spine's way of chilling out. Standing or sitting in one position for a long time inevitably channels all the stresses through one area of your spine, so that one set of joints, ligaments, muscles and tendons has to do all the work. Eventually they will tire and at that point you need to change position to give that set of spinal structures a rest and get another lot to take over. So during your long-haul flight you need to change position often. Keep this in mind and:
- Have the seat back upright for a while, then put it in recline for a while.
- Use a cushion or a pillow to support your lower back

most of the time, but occasionally remove it and sit back against the seat for twenty minutes. Sit on it for a while to raise your pelvis, then use it to support your lumbar spine.

- Enjoy an occasional five-minute slump.
- Remove the pillow from your back and spend five minutes or so every hour doing the key circulation-boosting exercises shown on pages 92–4.
- Be nosy and check out the other passengers. Turn your upper body slowly and gently from the hips to see what is happening in the aisle, then turn back the other way before turning to the front again.
- Get out of your seat once every hour or so and walk along the aisle. Take the opportunity to stretch.
- Once every four hours, run through the complete exercise programme on pages 95–111. It will stretch your back, stretch all the ligaments, exercise all the muscle groups, and wake up the tendons.

Resting and sleeping

Most people want to sleep on a long-haul flight, but do bear in mind that sleeping in an uncomfortable position can be very stressful for your spine. It is also believed to increase the likelihood of blood clots developing in the leg veins. The upper spine and neck need to be a focus of attention when you sleep. If the headrest of the chair seems to push your head forwards, you need to support your upper spine and your neck with a cushion. If the seat back does not have side supports for your head, the pillow needs to be wide enough to prevent your head from lolling from side to side. Waking up with a pain in the neck is one of the discomforts of economy-class air travel. For this reason it is better not to sleep on a long-haul flight if you are travelling in economy class – fly during the day, when you are less likely to be sleepy. If you have to take a night flight book business class with an airline that advertises seats that convert into flat beds. If you travel premium economy with plenty of leg room, try to take short naps and get up and move about each time you wake up.

If you are sitting fairly upright your head is in danger of falling forwards, towards your chest. When this happens, watchful sensors in your neck detect the forward movement and speedily alert the brain, which interprets the movement as a sign of danger and wakes you up. One way of preventing this is to use one of the U-shaped pillows which are often sold at air terminals, and put it round the *front* of your neck so you rest your chin on it. It will also stop your head lolling to either side, especially if you encircle your neck with one or two pillows, so you may need to ask the cabin staff or to improvise. Follow this check list to prepare yourself to rest or for a nap while sitting upright:

1. Move your sacrum close up against the back of the chair and rest both your feet flat on the floor or, if you can, on a footrest.
2. Position a pillow or lumbar roll so that it supports your lumbar spine well.

3. Recline the seat, but not too far. If you can gauge it, an angle of up to 105° from the horizontal is about right.

4. Experiment with neck supports to find the most comfortable resting position.

5. If you want to sleep but find it difficult, try using eye shades and ear plugs.

CHAPTER FOUR
In-Flight Exercises

This whole chapter is devoted to exercises you can do while sitting in an aircraft seat. Some of you will be sitting in first class or business class, where you have plenty of room to move, but it is just as important for you to do these movements and stretches as it is for those passengers in economy class, whose space is more restricted. It is not natural for your body to sit still for many hours.

However, for those of you flying in the economy seats, where you are more confined, it is especially important to move and stretch and exercise as much as you can. The exercises in this chapter can be carried out in restricted space, and it will benefit you to lift your knees and raise your arms, even if you can only lift and raise them a little way. Use every opportunity you have to move. If you are sitting in an aisle seat, stretch your legs into the aisle now and again when no one is passing. If you are sitting by a window, take advantage of a neighbour's temporary absence to stretch your arms and legs outwards for a while. You will need to get out of your seat now and again just to visit the washroom, so use the time to stretch your legs and lift your feet up and down, to extend up to your full height, and to spread your arms out.

Start off with the five key exercises and the massage on pages 92–4. They need little space and take less than five minutes. They can be fun to do and they leave you with a satisfying feeling of getting your circulation going. Later, you might feel like working through the main programme, which starts on page

95. It exercises every part of your body from face to feet and leaves you feeling as if you have eased all the stiffness out of your joints and muscles.

It is very important not to sit without moving for a long time and then fall asleep in the same uncomfortable position, so these exercises and stretches are followed by sequences of breathing and relaxation techniques to relax you and perhaps help you sleep. If you exercise first and rest afterwards, you will wake up feeling much more refreshed and less cramped if you do happen to fall asleep. If you prefer not to sleep, perhaps to minimize jet lag at your destination, finish after the stretches. And later, when your flight is over, remember the stretches and relaxation sequence. They make a very effective pre-sleep routine which will help you sleep.

Self-massage techniques are an important part of these exercises. If it is carried out regularly, massage stimulates the circulation and relaxes the muscles. Many airlines offer face, head and shoulders, and foot massage to passengers awaiting their flights in the first-class lounges. This programme includes self-massage for the feet and legs, hands and arms, neck and shoulders, and the face. Self-massage is a therapeutic activity on a long flight and helps relieve stress if you are a nervous flier. Some passengers report that it

However roomy and comfortable your seat you still need to spend time exercising your legs and feet on a long flight.

seems to reduce jet lag, especially if it is followed up with a full body massage as soon as possible after arriving at the destination.

What will the neighbours say?

Only a year or two ago the idea of exercising in mid-flight was so novel that the passenger who first tested these exercises was a little nervous of how neighbours would react to spinal arching, vigorous leg massage and rhythmic foot-tapping. But no one in a crowded economy cabin so much as noticed a neighbour making unusual movements and we can report with some confidence that you need not feel shy about doing these exercises in public.

On a second trial they were tested in first class, where passengers proved more curious about their neighbour's unusual movements. Since those trial flights, however, doctors, aviation health organizations and airlines have launched publicity campaigns to alert everyone to the dangers of sitting in cramped conditions for hours without moving. Now, airlines show exercise videos and publish exercise routines in their in-flight magazines to encourage passengers to stretch and move about when flying long-haul. So, whether your seat is in the nose of the aircraft or the tail, you are now likely to be one of many passengers exercising healthily in mid-flight.

But one person of several who have tried out these exercises on long-haul flights in recent months reported a few glances from neighbours in economy class, and that would be enough to deter some people from trying them out. If you are one of the many people who especially dislike exercising in public, be reassured that even invisible movements will help boost your circulation. Lifting and lowering your toes and heels, stretching your spine up and your arms out to your knees, tightening and releasing the muscles of your stomach, buttocks, thighs, legs and arms, raising and lowering your shoulders, and turning your head from side to side will all help your circulation and release the muscular tension caused by prolonged immobility. For these movements to be really effective, you will have to repeat them all a few times in succession and run through them at least once an hour while airborne.

Many of the exercises shown in this chapter involve minimal movement, so the people around you will not realize you are exercising.

Key circulation-boosters

The short sequence of five key exercises are designed to prevent traveller's DVT. They consist of rhythmic movements and massage techniques to stop the blood circulation from slowing and getting sluggish, and they will keep the lymph flowing around its separate circulation network, enabling it to continue its important role in maintaining your body's immune system. To have these effects, however, these key exercises must be performed at least once every hour you are awake during the flight.

Main exercise sequence

The main programme consists of light movements and exercises in four parts, and it takes about half an hour. It needs to be carried out at least once every four hours. The first part of the programme consists of exercises and massage techniques which work together to give the blood and lymph circulation a vigorous boost. These movements also exercise all the major joints, preventing stiffness; they stretch the spine from tail to neck, relieving pressure on the lower back; and they stress and relax the major muscle groups to lift tension. Do them slowly and thoughtfully. Never rush an exercise session. If something interrupts you, just relax, deal with the matter, sit and breathe deeply for a few seconds to restore your concentration, then continue where you left off. Try to exercise rhythmically, because rhythmic movements stimulate the circulation most effectively.

To be effective, in-flight exercises need to be carried out at regular intervals while you are airborne.

Stretch and relax

Travelling can be very stressful, particularly so for the 25 per cent of us who dislike air travel, but if you progress to 'stretch and relax' – the second part of the programme – you will find those feelings of tension and stress ebb away from body and mind. Stretching is a marvellous way of relaxing, and these exercises stretch and rotate every moveable part of your body, from neck and shoulders to ankles and feet. They end with an energetic tap dance which exercises your concentration and is as invigorating as a brisk walk.

Deep breathing

The breathing exercises are especially effective for neutralizing anxiety and helping you relax mentally. At the same time, breathing increases the supply of oxygen to the blood, the brain, and the tissues, so it has a mildly stimulating effect on the circulation. It also helps your body adapt to the low air pressure in the cabin. These exercises combine rhythmic breathing with tightening and relaxing the muscles, and the two actions combine to stimulate circulation still more. As you breathe out, you let the tension go more completely each time. For this reason, try the breathing exercises out, even if the people around you are making a lot of noise. You may find that by the end you will have relaxed so much that the disturbance has receded into the background.

If you are travelling in economy class and your legs are very cramped it is better not to sleep because sleeping in a cramped position encourages traveller's DVT. However, flying is tiring and you may drop off despite yourself. If this happens, get up as soon

as you wake up and walk down the aisle to the washroom, stretch your legs, and run through the five key
circulation-booster exercises.

Deep relaxation

If you are flying in business or first class where the
seats recline into flat beds, this part of the programme
is especially effective on a night flight. Eventually
most other passengers quieten down, and you may
find that the stretching, breathing and relaxation help
you drift off to sleep.

Visualization exercises, a fail-safe relaxation technique first discovered in the ancient East and since
rediscovered time and again, complete the programme.
These exercises and stretches and this massage, combined with deep relaxation, can leave you feeling completely relaxed. And if you are a frequent flier who
finds it hard to sleep, use this programme to help yourself deal with the effects of jet lag. You may even find
it a good way of relaxing whenever stress and tension
prevent you from achieving a good night's sleep,
whether or not you are flying.

When to exercise

Ideally, these exercises need to be done once every four
hours to keep your circulation healthy during a long
flight. But use them to make yourself more comfortable at any time during a flight. If take-off makes you
nervous, relieve the tension by breathing and stretch-

ing while the aircraft waits for take-off. Exercise to dissipate stiffness after watching a film, or after drifting off into a light sleep. On night flights it is good to run through the exercises after eating and before settling down to sleep – the programme is especially relaxing when you can be quiet and uninterrupted as you work through it.

Aids to exercise

As we write, many new devices are appearing on the market, designed to help passengers exercise in-flight. A massage stick or a rolled towel or scarf are excellent for massaging the legs. You grip one end of the stick or the towel with each hand and pull it up the back of the leg or along the back of the thigh. It gives a deeper massage than you can manage with your fingers, and your hands do not tire so quickly. Exercise aids such as the Stepfit and the Airogym (see page 49) can also make the leg and feet exercises still more effective, because they resist the action of the feet, making them work harder. If your feet do not reach the floor easily, the inflated Airogym will give you a raised base on which to stand, and a clean surface on which to rest bare feet.

So, whether you are a seasoned traveller or on your first long-haul flight, take time to read through these exercises and absorb them, ready to start. Take your time over the movements. It may be a while since you spent some prime time with yourself; now is an excellent opportunity. Make the most of it and enjoy it.

If you are wearing earrings, rings, bracelets, or a wrist watch, take them off carefully, wrap them a handkerchief, and put them in your pocket or your bag. If you are wearing a belt, loosen it, and ease any tight clothes. Take off your shoes and, if you wish, your socks. Are you too hot? If so, ask for some iced water to drink. Your seat needs to be in the upright position and the seat belt only loosely fastened (bear in mind that all airlines advise passengers to keep their seat belts fastened even during cruising, in case of sudden turbulence).

If you are reclining against a loose cushion or a foam support, remove it before exercising. Later, when you come to the relaxation exercises, you can replace it if you wish, and put the seat back if it will recline. When you are ready to begin, sit upright, your feet on the floor, or on a support if they do not reach the floor.

Just before you begin, direct your awareness to the space between you and your neighbour(s). Use that space as well as you can, taking care not to encroach on a neighbour's space accidentally as you move your elbows, shoulders, legs, or feet.

KEY CIRCULATION-BOOSTERS

The five key exercises on pages 92–94 are important for boosting your blood circulation and preventing blood clots from developing in your veins. Perform them once an hour while you are awake, more often if you feel like it. Don't miss them, especially if it is difficult for you to get out of your seat once every hour or so to walk along the cabin and back. You should also do them if you intend to sleep, and again when you wake up.

Even if you are tall and your seat gives you little leg room, you should still have room to do almost all of these exercises. If you have long legs and you are sitting in economy class you may be unable to lift your legs to massage them. Sitting in such restricted space makes massage all the more important for you, so spend two minutes massaging during your next visit to the toilet. Repeat the exercises one to four times in succession, working up a rhythm.

WARNING

These exercises are suitable for most people, but if you have a replacement hip or suffer from high blood pressure or heart problems, do not do them without first checking with your doctor. If you are on medication for any condition you should also check with a doctor whether any of the exercises are unsuitable for you. Passengers with a medical condition need only avoid the movement exercises. The breathing and relaxation can cause no harm and can be done by anyone, and the massage is gentle and safe unless you have a wound or an injury at the site of the massage.

1 TREADMILL

Sit upright, and move your seat deep into the back of the chair. Press your toes down on to the floor and raise your heels. Press down with your toes while counting slowly to six, and rest. Repeat six times.

2 FOOT ROTATIONS

Right foot: lift your right thigh off the chair and clasp your hands together beneath it to support your leg. Rotate your foot inwards slowly, counting to six ... then change direction, circling your foot outwards. Repeat, circling inwards and then outwards, trying to draw a perfect circle with your toes. Release your right leg.

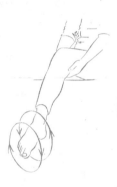

Left foot: lift your left thigh, clasp your hands under it, behind the knee, and rotate your left foot outwards to a count of six, then inwards to a count of six. Repeat, release your thigh and rest. Now repeat the whole exercise six to ten times.

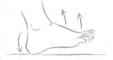

3 ANKLE STRETCHES

Place your feet flat on the floor, about 6 inches (15 centimetres) apart. Push your heels down against the floor and lift your toes as high as you can off the floor, so your foot points upwards and the ankle hinges back. Hold for a moment, then relax. Repeat five more times ... and rest.

4 TOE PRESSES

You can do this exercise wearing shoes if they are soft and roomy. If not, it is better to take off your shoes.

Spread your toes and wiggle them, as if you are paddling on a sandy shore and digging them into the soft sand. Press them down to make the sand squash up between your toes. Relax, then repeat three times. Now curl your toes inwards, raising the arches of your feet ... and rest. Repeat the exercise six to ten times.

5 LEG MASSAGE

Right leg: lift your right foot and rest it lightly on top of the left one, so your right thigh is lifted off the seat. First, pummel your calf muscles with your fingers, down to your ankle if you can reach, then bunch the fingers of each hand together and draw them up your 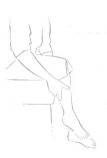 leg from ankle to knee, stopping to knead as you go. Move your fingers round to your shin and massage upwards. Finally, if your clothes allow, massage the back of your thigh from the knee towards your body. Repeat three times.

Left leg: put your right foot on the floor, lift your

left leg and rest it lightly on top of your right foot. Repeat, massaging your left calf, shin, and thigh.

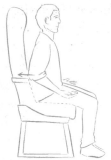

FINISH WITH A STRETCH
First: put both feet flat on the floor and push your seat against the back of the chair. Bend your arms, press your elbows against your sides, and turn your palms up. Now press your elbows against the chair back, to make your shoulder blades move inwards towards your spine. Repeat five times ... then rest.

Second: put the palms of your hands together and lift them up front as high as you can, then lift your shoulders and pull them down. Raise your shoulders again, while stretching your back and arching it. Repeat five times, and rest.

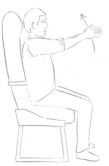

EXERCISE PROGRAMME

Wherever you are seated in the aircraft, whatever your age or sex, you should do this sequence of exercises at least once during your flight. They are essential for your health, and they will make you feel much more comfortable. If you are tall or have long legs and you are hemmed in by other seats, you may find it difficult to do some exercises, but try to find a way. The leg and foot exercises are especially important for you if your leg room is restricted. This programme also contains essential exercises for your back, and it works your neck and shoulders, where tension often resides. All parts of the body work together, so it is best not to pick and choose exercises, but rather to work through the exercises in order, thinking about each part of the body in turn.

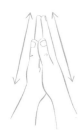

MASSAGE YOUR HANDS

If you are inactive for a long time, the flow of blood to your hands may slow, starving the tissues of nutrients and warmth. The next two exercises stimulate blood flow and stretch the many small joints of the hands and fingers.

- Put the palms and fingers of your hands together and rub them forwards and back, forwards and back.
- Interlace your fingers and tease them forwards and back to massage between the fingers. If your left thumb is on top and your right little finger at the

bottom, release your fingers and interlock them again with the right thumb on top and the left little finger at 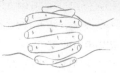 the bottom, and tease the fingers forwards and back to massage them.

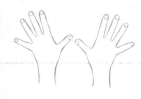

STRETCH YOUR FINGERS

- Release your fingers and stretch them out, counting slowly one ... and ... two ... and ... three ... and ... four ... and ... five ... and ... six ... and rest.
- Make a fist with each hand and hold while counting to six.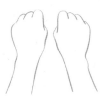
- Repeat: stretch the fingers to a count of six, clench the fists to a count of six ... and rest.

ROTATE YOUR WRISTS

We rarely exercise our hands, yet we need to keep them flexible. Take this opportunity to stretch and flex the wrist joints in every direction.

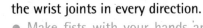

- Make fists with your hands and circle them inwards from the wrists. Follow with five more circles, trying to make them perfectly even.
- Repeat, this time circling outwards from the wrist.

MASSAGE YOUR FOREARMS

This is a very effective massage to stimulate blood flow along the arms. You need to grip your arms firmly, but not so hard that you end up with bruises. If you have been lifting and carrying heavy bags you will soothe your arm muscles with this vigorous massage.

● Release your right fist. If you have long sleeves, push or roll them up to the elbow. Then hold your left wrist in front of you and clasp it firmly but gently with your right hand.

● Now twist your left wrist back-wards and forwards inside the gripping right fingers and thumb of your right hand. As you twist, move your right hand slowly up your left arm to just above the elbow, then move back down to the wrist.

Twist backwards and forwards. Grip firmly

● Repeat, then release your hands ... and rest.

● Make a fist with your right hand, clasp your right wrist with your left hand, and twist your right wrist backwards and forwards.

● Repeat, then release your right hand ... and rest.

WORK YOUR RIGHT ELBOW

Ever thought of exercising your elbows? These two joints work tirelessly through the day, taking the strain. Here is your chance to reward them with some quality time. If your seat adjoins another, take care not to biff your neighbour: do not let your fists stray outwards

past your shoulders.

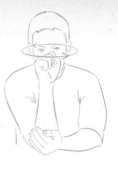

- Make a fist with your right hand, then bend your right arm in front of you so the fist is in front of your face. Now cup your left palm around your right elbow. Keeping the elbow still, draw a circle in the air with your right fist, moving it out to the right, round to the left, and in towards you. Draw three more circles, then change direction, circling out to the left, round to the right and in towards you, four times.

- Repeat, circling four times to the right and four times to the left. Then release your fist ... and rest.

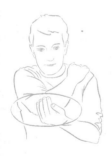

LOOSEN YOUR RIGHT SHOULDER

This self-massage will release tension in your shoulders. Keep your body still as you move your arm, letting your hand slide over your shoulder and move freely around. Take care not to annoy your neighbour by pulling your elbow too far out.

- Put your open right hand on your left shoulder, then cup your left palm around your right elbow. Pull the elbow round in a circle with your left hand, moving it inwards, to the left, then down, and out to the right as far as your shoulder, and up. Draw three more circles, then change direction, circling out, down, in, and up.

● Repeat, circling inwards four times, and outwards four times, then rest.

MASSAGE YOUR RIGHT SIDE
This is a massage to soothe your neck and your shoulder joints if they ache from carrying heavy luggage. If you find a tight spot as you massage, work on it for a while to ease the tension.

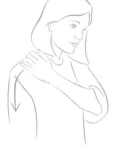

● Slip your left hand around the right side of your neck and draw your fingers towards the heel of your hand, pressing firmly but gently to massage your neck in a stroking motion. Do this a few times, then work down your neck and along your right shoulder.

WORK YOUR LEFT ELBOW
Now repeat the last three exercises, this time on the left side of your body, so here are the exercises again for the left side:

● Make a fist with your left hand, then bend your left arm in front of you so the fist is in front of your face. Cup your right palm around your left elbow. Keeping the elbow still, draw a circle in the air with your left fist, moving it out to the left, round to the right, and in towards you. Draw three more circles, then change direction, circling out to the right, round to the left and in towards you, four times.

- Repeat, circling four times to the left and four times to the right. Then release your fist ... and rest.

LOOSEN YOUR LEFT SHOULDER

- Put your open left hand on your right shoulder, then cup your right palm around your left elbow. Pull the elbow round in a circle with your right hand, moving it inwards, to the right, then down, out to the left as far as your shoulder, and up. Draw three more circles, then change direction, circling out, down, in, and up.
- Repeat, circling inwards four times, and outwards four times. Then rest.

MASSAGE YOUR LEFT SIDE

- Slip your right hand around the left side of your neck and draw your fingers towards the heel of your hand, pressing firmly but gently, to massage your neck in a stroking motion. Do this a few times, then work down your neck and along your left shoulder.

WORK THE TREADLE

This is a very important exercise because contracting the calf muscles rhythmically pumps the blood out of the lower legs, where it tends to pool when you sit upright and immobile, giving clots a chance to form.

- Place the heels and toes of both feet on the floor, sit upright, and move your seat deep into the back of the chair. Imagine pushing down the treadle of an old house organ or sewing machine with your feet: press your toes into the floor and raise your heels into the air. Press while counting slowly to six, then rest.

● Now put your hands on your knees and repeat the exercise, pressing your hands down on your knees to resist their upward movement. Push down slowly and strongly with your toes while raising your heels, and as you do so, sit deeper into the chair seat. Press while counting slowly to six ... then rest.

TIGHTEN UP

Just tightening and releasing the major muscle groups stimulates circulation, because the muscle action exerts a pumping action on surrounding veins. This exercise stimulates the flow of blood along the thighs and abdomen to the heart. It also tenses and strengthens the pelvic floor – the hammock of muscles that lies across the lower part of the abdomen and surrounds the urethra and the anus.

● Work the treadle (above) once more, and this time draw your lower stomach muscles up and in towards your lower back. At the same time, lift your spine from tail to the top of your neck, stretching it up. Tighten the muscles of your thighs and buttocks as you push against the

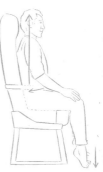

floor, and hold, counting to six. Relax ... and repeat
six times, holding for a slow count of six each time.

MASSAGE YOUR LEGS

Your calves and thighs need to be massaged strongly,
so press the fingers of both hands tightly together and
draw them firmly up your leg and along your thigh,
pressing your fingers into the muscles as they move.
Alternatively, hold the ends of a folded towel in each
hand, press the towel against your leg, and draw it
firmly upwards. A wooden or plastic massage stick may
be used in the same way. It gives a deeper massage
than the hands, which tend to tire quickly. Massage
upwards, towards the heart.

- Start with both feet flat on the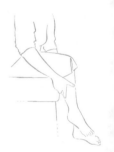
  floor, then lift your right foot
  and rest it lightly on top of the
  left one, so your right thigh is
  off the seat. Pummel your calf
  muscles with your fingers right
  down to your ankle, if you can
  reach. If you notice any tight
  spots, concentrate on massaging them until they ease.
- Massage your calf firmly from the ankle to the knee,
  then move your fingers round to your shin and massage upwards.
- Now, if your clothes allow, massage the back of the
  thigh from the knee back towards your body.
- Place your right foot on the floor, then lift your left
  leg and rest it lightly on top of your right foot to lift

the thigh off the seat, and massage your left thigh, calf, and shin.

MASSAGE YOUR FEET
These movements exercise the toes and the arches of the feet. They are best done with bare feet, so if you can and if you have not already done so, take off your shoes and hosiery. Your feet need to be flat on the floor, so rest them on a newspaper or a cushion. It is possible to do this exercise wearing shoes if they are soft and roomy.

- Spread your toes and wiggle them, as if you are paddling on a sandy shore, digging them into the soft sand. Now press them down to make the sand squash up between your toes.
- Relax, then repeat, spreading your toes and moving them in the sand. Now squash the sand through your toes twice more.
- Curl your toes strongly inwards, raising the arches of your feet ... and rest.

STRETCH YOUR ANKLES
This circulation exercise will send blood coursing upwards from your feet on its return journey along the veins of your legs to your heart. It is most effective if performed strongly and rhythmically. It also exercises the complex ankle joints and stretches the muscles and tendons of the feet and lower legs.

- Place your feet flat on the floor, about 15 centimetres (6 inches) apart. Push your heels down against the floor and lift your 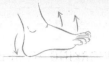 toes as high as you can off the floor, so your foot points upwards and the ankle hinges back. Hold for a moment ... then relax.
- Repeat the exercise with both feet five more times ... and rest.

MASSAGE YOUR HEAD AND NECK
Soothe any tension remaining in the complex muscle structure of your face by massaging your forehead and temples. Before rotating your head at the end, lift your spine from the tailbone to the crown of your head.

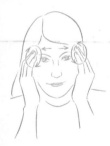

- Place the tips of your fingers against your temples and massage gently and rhythmically with a circular motion.
- Move your fingers to your forehead, rest your fingertips above your eyebrows, and massage gently, making small circles with your fingers. Then massage outwards to the temples, and finish by stroking your eyebrows outwards.

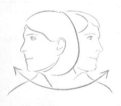

- Holding your head upright, turn it slowly to the right to look over your right shoulder, then rotate it to the front, and turn it to look over your left shoulder. Repeat twice ... then rest.

WORKING YOUR BACK MUSCLES

This exercise works on the upper spine, stretching and bending to release any tiredness resulting from poor posture. If you do not have room to stretch your hands out in front of you in the second part of the exercise, bend your elbows and raise your arms as high as you can while you lift and lower your shoulders.

● Sit with your feet on the floor and your seat against the back of the chair, place your forearms and elbows against your sides, and turn the palms up. Now press your elbows back against the chair to make the muscles between your shoulder blades move inwards, towards your spine. Repeat five times ... then relax.

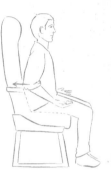

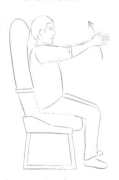

● Put the palms of your hands together and lift them up in front as high as you can, then lift your shoulders, and drop them. Lift your shoulders again, stretch and arch your back, then drop your shoulders ... and rest.

FINISH

Complete the sequence by shaking your hands and fingers lightly for a few seconds, as if you are playing the maracas ... then rest.

Stretch and relax

In our minds physical action and relaxation tend to go hand in hand. Relaxation is often associated with playing games in the park, perhaps, or on the beach. Being active gives you a chance to relax. The activity does not have to be so vigorous, however. These stretches are enough to enable you to relax afterwards.

STRETCH LIKE A CAT

This exercise stretches the whole body in stages, beginning with the arms in step 1. If you can, stretch your arms out in front, but if the seat in front blocks the movement, stretch them downwards, towards your knees. Work slowly, giving your back a satisfying stretch in step 2. In step 3, feel your buttock muscles contract as you push down. Press the feet equally inwards, and down against the floor. If your legs do not quite reach the floor and you have nothing to rest them on, just push down on your toes.

Step 1

● Sit upright with both feet flat on the floor. Interlace your fingers to clasp your hands together, then turn them over so the palms face outwards, away from you, and stretch your arms out in front or down towards your knees. Bring your hands back towards your chest, turning the palms to face you. Repeat ... then relax.

Step 2

- Interlace your fingers, turn your palms to face outwards, and stretch your arms out, then curve your shoulders and back like a cat stretching, pushing back against the chair seat.
- Sit upright, separating your hands and turning the palms upwards, and press your elbows back against the chair, pushing your spine away from the chair back. Hold for a few seconds ... then relax.

Step 3

- Interlace your fingers, turn your palms outwards, stretch your arms, and curve your shoulders and back, then sit upright, keeping your arms and interlinked hands stretching forwards. Now press both feet together and down against the floor, and hold while you count slowly to six.

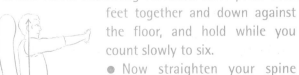

  - Now straighten your spine so you sit upright like an Egyptian statue. Hold for a count of six ... then relax.
  - Repeat step 3 twice ... then rest.

ROTATE YOUR FEET

This exercise works the ankle joints, so rotate your feet from the ankles, not your leg from the knee.

- Lift your left thigh off the chair and support some of the leg weight by clasping your hands under the thigh just behind the knee. Let your left foot hang freely from the ankle.

- Rotate your foot to the left, then round to the right and back to the left, counting slowly to six. Imagine your toes are a brush painting a perfectly even circle in the air.

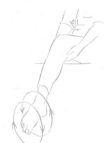

- Now change direction, rotating your foot to the right and paint a perfect, even circle in the air with your toes, counting slowly to six.

- Now repeat, circling your foot to the left and then to the right. Then unclasp your hands and rest your left thigh on the chair.

- Now lift the right thigh off the chair, clasp your hands under it, just behind the knee, and rotate your right foot to the right to a count of six. Change direction, rotating to the left to a count of six, then to the right, then to the left again.

- Unclasp your hands and rest your right thigh back on the chair seat.

ROTATE YOUR SHOULDERS

This exercise works the shoulder joint by rotating it rhythmically.

- Sit upright and lift your shoulders as if someone were pulling them up to your ears, then rotate them smoothly back and down. Rotate a second time up ... back ... and down, and a third time up ... back ... and down. Rest and repeat.

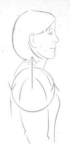

TIGHTEN YOUR HAMSTRINGS

You might have to lean forwards slightly to do this exercise, and if your feet do not touch the floor, you may need to lift your heels. Pressing and resisting tightens the hamstrings at the backs of your thighs and your buttocks. Do not let your shoulders move forwards – keep them open and broad.

- Still sitting upright, move your feet together. Straighten your hands and fingers, place the palms together, and rest your joined hands between your knees.

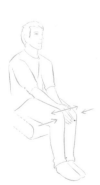

Hands push out
Knees push in

- Press your heels together gently, and push outwards with your hands while pressing your knees inwards with equal pressure against your hands. Hold, sitting tall, while counting slowly to six ... and relax.
- Repeat: press heels together and push outwards with hands and inwards with knees, tightening hamstrings and buttocks. Hold for a count of six, sitting tall, keeping

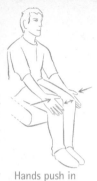

your shoulders broad, and relaxing your neck and head. Relax ... repeat for a third time ... and rest.

- Now put one hand on the outside of each knee, press heels together, tighten buttocks, and this time press the knees outwards, resisting their push with your hands while counting to six. Repeat three times ... then rest.

Hands push in
Knees push out

DO A TAP DANCE
Practise this exercise until you can do it rhythmically, like a dance. It will reinforce your circulatory systems and relax you, body and mind.

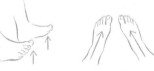

up and ...   ... in and tap ...

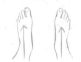

... and centre and tap ...

... and up and out and tap ...

- Move your feet 15 centimetres (6 inches) apart, press your heels down on the floor, and lift up your forefeet and toes.
- Now practise the sequence: swivel both feet towards each other a little, and tap the toes on the floor; lift the forefeet, swivel them outwards a little so the toes point straight ahead, and tap on the floor; lift the forefeet, turn them out, away from each other, and tap on the floor; then lift

the forefeet, swivel them inwards so they point ahead, and tap on the floor.

- Now repeat: lift the forefeet ... turn them in, and tap ... lift the forefeet ... turn them back to the centre, and tap ... lift the forefeet ... turn them out, and tap ... lift the forefeet ... turn them back to the centre, and tap.
- Repeat several times, getting a rhythm going.
- When your calf muscles tire, press your toes down against the floor, lift your heels and pump them up and down six times.
- Continue tapping: up ... and in and tap ... and up ... and centre and tap ... and up ... and out and tap ... and up ... and centre and tap ... When your calves tire again, stop ... and rest.

Deep breathing

Muscle exertion combined with breathing is a powerful relaxant and prepares the body and the mind for rest. Keep your chair in the upright position. Have your seat belt fastened but slightly loosened, and press both feet against the floor to move yourself deep into the back of your seat. If at any time you want to stop following the programme, stretch the arms as in step 1 of 'stretch like a cat' on page 106: lace your fingers, turn your palms out, and stretch your arms towards your knees.

Your back is now comfortably supported. Rest your forearms on your lap with the palms turned down, and rest the back of your head gently against the headrest. Read through each exercise first, then close your eyes to do it, concentrating on your breathing until the noise around you becomes a background hum.

PLAY THE FLUTE

Breathe in deeply and rhythmically in this exercise, to relax completely. Experience the difference between holding your breath for an instant as you finish each in-breath, and letting go slowly and relaxing completely on each out-breath.

- Start by breathing slowly in and out, in and out, in and out. In through the nose, out through the mouth. In through the nose, out through the mouth. Breathe out so evenly that you imagine blowing into a flute and playing the purest and most perfect note in a valley surrounded by echoing mountains. When you finish your next in-breath, hold your breath for a moment to listen for the echo of that golden note.

- Breathe out again, blowing evenly into the flute to play the same note, letting your breath escape slowly until the note fades and dies away. Then breathe in through the nose again and wait ... holding your breath to listen for the echo.

- Repeat three times, breathing evenly out through the mouth to let that golden note sound until it dies away, then breathing in through the nose and holding your breath to listen for the echo. Repeat a few more times.

CLENCH AND LET GO

This exercise emphasizes the difference between tension and relaxation. Feel your whole body tense, and then relax as you release the tension on the out-breath.

- Breathe in through the nose and hold your breath while clenching your left fist and pressing your left arm tight against your body. Wait, breathing suspended, listening for the echo of the golden note, then breathe out slowly, letting the tension go completely, unclenching your fist and letting your hand rest in your lap.

- Repeat the exercise: breathe in ... and wait, clench fist, tighten arm ... wait and listen ... then release. Repeat once more, then rest.

- Breathe in and hold ... suspending the breath while clenching your right fist and pressing your right arm tight against your body. Wait ... listen for the echo of the golden note ... then breathe out slowly, letting the tension go completely ... unclenching your fist and letting your right hand rest in your lap.

- Repeat twice ... and rest.

TIGHTEN UP AND LET GO

- Now press the palms of your hands together, and as you do so press your elbows against your sides and tighten your arm muscles. Sit upright and stretch up tall, then rest.

- Breathe in and hold ... suspending your breath as you press the palms of your hands together, press your elbows against your sides, and tighten your arm muscles. Wait ... then breathe out slowly and evenly, and let go completely ... relax your neck muscles ... relax your arms ... and let your hands fall to your lap.

- Repeat four times ... and rest.

PULL OUT AND LET GO

- This time, hook the fingers of your left hand to those of your right hand. Breathe in and hold ... suspending your breathing ... pulling your hooked fingers in opposite directions as you listen for the echo of the golden note. Then breathe out slowly and evenly ... and let go completely ... relaxing your neck muscles ...unhook your fingers to let your hands fall to your lap.

- Repeat four times ... and rest.

PRESS AND RESIST

- Put your hands on the outsides of your knees, breathe in through the nose, and hold ... suspending your breathing as you press your knees into your hands and your hands into your knees. Press and resist, tighten your thigh muscles ... and listen for the echo of the golden note ... then breathe out through the mouth and let go completely ... relax your thigh muscles.

- Repeat twice ... then place your hands on your lap and rest for a while ... breathe in and out rhythmically and peacefully.

- Place your palms against the insides of your knees, breathe in through the nose ... and hold, suspending your breathing as you press your knees into your hands and your hands into your knees. Press and resist, tighten your thigh muscles ... then breathe out slowly through the mouth ... let go completely ... relax your thigh muscles.
- Repeat twice, then put your hands on your lap ... and relax.

Deep relaxation

Now you can rest. Read through these last instructions, then set the book aside, recline the aircraft seat and relax back into it. Relax your head against the headrest, close your eyes, and see your body as it is now, comfortable and relaxed, perhaps ready to sleep.

- I see in my mind ... my hands ... relaxed, my arms ... relaxed, my legs and my feet ... relaxed. I think of my shoulders and neck ... and I relax the muscles completely. I think of the muscles in my face ... and relax them ... I relax my eyes ... and my tongue and throat. My back is comfortable, supported by the chair ... I relax and lengthen it ... my shoulders feel open, broad and relaxed. Now, I can enjoy this state of relaxation. I can continue to rest ... I imagine being in my favourite spot ... lying on soft grass ... listening to bird song ... lying in golden sunlight on warm sands ... listening to the sound of the sea ... I might just gently drift into sleep ...

Wake up

Later, as you wake, count one, two, three, and stretch your arms out forwards. Open your eyes and return to your surroundings, then sit up.

CHAPTER FIVE
Travelling Under Pressure

Your jetliner climbs just above 10,700 metres (about 35,000 feet) and relaxes into cruise mode, engines settling into a steady hum. You read, watch a video, exercise, eat a meal. The cabin is warm, perhaps a little stuffy. Outside, there is much less air about. Gravity compresses the envelope of atmosphere surrounding the Earth, so that close to sea level it is about four times more dense than at jet cruising levels. Climbers on the peak of Mount Everest need oxygen to breathe, and jets cruise about 2 kilometres – more than a mile higher. At those altitudes the air may be as cold as –55° Celsius.

For all these reasons the systems that keep an aircraft cabin pressurized, aerated and warm are far more complex than the air-conditioning that heats and cools your home and workplace. Their job is to make the cabin environment habitable. In the half-century since passenger aircraft began flying at high altitudes, this complex of life-support systems has proved its reliability: passengers do not worry that the air they are breathing might unexpectedly give out, or that the temperatures might drop below freezing. Yet passengers in economy class often complain of stale air, and cabin air quality always heads the list of complaints after long-haul flights. What is wrong with the air in high-flying jets, and why don't the airlines do something to improve it?

The next two chapters explore the effects on health of the systems that make the cabin environment habitable, from pressurization to air-conditioning. They explain current controversies surrounding passenger health and comfort, and suggest things you can do to improve your personal portion of the cabin environment, and reduce the risk of in-flight illness.

Thin air

Jetliners cruise at 9,100–12,200 metres (30,000–40,000 feet). At these altitudes the outside air contains 21 per cent oxygen, the same proportion as the air on the ground, but the air is thinner. The higher you climb, the lower the air pressure – the total force of gases pressing down on the Earth – so at progressively higher altitudes each breath of air contains fewer molecules of oxygen. For an aircraft to fly at 10,700 metres (35,000 feet), the air inside it has to be at a high enough pressure for people to be able to absorb enough oxygen from it through breathing.

So when aircraft engineers are designing a new commercial jet, they have to make its whole structure strong enough for the air pressure inside to be higher than the pressure of the outside air. You would expect them to make its internal pressure equivalent to the air pressure at sea level, because the human body works most efficiently at that level, but from an engineering point of view, this poses problems.

A jet with an internal pressure equivalent to sea level would need a very strong structure. Concorde, which flies at 15,200–18,300 metres (50,000–60,000 feet) where the air pressure is twenty times less dense than at sea level, has a costly steel and titanium structure, whereas most aircraft are built from lighter, cheaper materials. Like Concorde, this high-strength jet would have to be small, with tiny windows. Concorde weighs almost as much as the Airbus A310, yet it carries half the number of passengers. Similarly, a jet featuring sea-level pressurization would be impracticably heavy, and it would burn similarly high quantities of fuel. All these factors would send ticket prices soaring way above Concorde rates.

Balancing the practicalities of designing the airframe against the needs of the human body and the costs of operating commercial jets, the aircraft industry settled on compromises. Most commercial jets can be pressurized up to a maximum of 3,000 metres (10,000 feet) above sea level, although in practice, internal cabin pressure rarely, if ever, rises that high. And they have to able to maintain a cabin pressure equivalent to a height of 2,400 metres (8,000 feet), however high they fly. That is the industry standard, accepted world-wide.

Aircraft pressurization is automatic, controlled by sensors and valves so that it remains constant through the aircraft, and during climb and descent the pressure changes gradually, in steps. However, it is adjustable within safe limits from the flight deck, and pilots normally set it at the equivalent of 1,800–2,100 metres (6,000–7,000 feet) for maximum passenger comfort. But such a low pressurization has a cost, in that the engines burn more fuel, so if pilots need to save fuel –

to respond to their airline's policy, perhaps – they will raise the pressure to 2,400 metres (8,000 feet). US Federal Aviation Administration regulations do not permit cabin pressure to exceed this level, but the British Civil Aviation Authority permits it when pilots need to fly high to avoid turbulent weather and other unexpected conditions. Recent studies have recorded occasions when pressure rose towards the equivalent of 2,700 metres (9,000 feet).

The effects of low air pressure

Humans live at astonishing altitudes. The highest human dwellings, according to *The Guinness Book of Records*, are in Basisi, in northern India, close to the Tibet border, at 5,988 metres (19,700 feet) high. But people who live at very high altitudes develop many adaptations to help them survive lower air pressure. They automatically breathe more deeply, for example, and they have more red blood cells, which carry oxygen. These adjustments take time, however, and passengers do not stay in an aircraft long enough for the body to adapt.

What happens in the body when pressure reduces is that the blood circulating through the lungs absorbs less oxygen. This is normally unnoticeable when the cabin is pressurized to around 1,800–2,100 metres (6,000–7,000 feet). At that altitude the amount of oxygen you take in with each breath is about 80 per cent of an in-breath at sea level, and the amount of oxygen dissolved in your blood is about 97 per cent of normal blood oxygen at sea level. In fact, many people live their lives breathing air whose pressure is well below what is normal for the rest of us. The usual operating pressure of a Boeing 747 cabin is the norm for everyone who lives in Mexico City, built 2,360 metres (7,200 feet) above sea level.

The lungs and blood circulation are so efficient that a healthy body can function well and shows few physical effects after a few hours in a cabin pressurized as high as 3,000 metres (10,000 feet). However, anyone suffering from the conditions listed below may experience some discomfort and may need extra oxygen at cruising altitude.

Supplementary oxygen has to be provided by the airline, but you must request it when booking your ticket, and you may be asked to pay for its supply. You will have to show confirmation from a physician that you need the oxygen, so give yourself plenty of time to make all the arrangements. Rather than take heavy oxygen cylinders on board, some airlines arrange for passengers to use the aircraft's reserve oxygen. Not all airlines will agree to fly passengers who need supplementary oxygen, so you may need to shop around.

Lowered concentrations of oxygen in the blood may cause headache, unsteadiness and sometimes nausea. People in the following risk categories must consult a physician before deciding to take any trip that involves flying for more than an hour. For long-haul flights they may need extra oxygen:

- **People with lung disease**, such as chronic bronchitis and emphysema.
- **Anyone who suffers from cardiovascular illness**, such as heart failure or heart disease.
- **The elderly:** from the age of fifty the concentration of oxygen in the blood is increasingly affected by cabin pressure. Healthy people in their fifties and sixties need not worry, but consult a physician specializing in aviation medicine if you are unsure.
- **Asthmatics:** people who have asthma attacks should consult their physician before flying and pack prescribed asthma inhalers and bronchodilators with them in their hand luggage. It is comforting to know that many irritants that cause asthma are automatically filtered out of the cabin air throughout the flight, so attacks may occur less frequently or with less severity during the flight.
- **Anyone with anaemia** – reduced numbers of red blood cells.

Smokers

Despite the fact that smoking was permitted on all airlines until the late-1980s and some have never banned it, smoking and flying in a pressurized jet do not go together. Smoking reduces the oxygen level of the blood to roughly the levels you experience in a pressurized aircraft cabin, so when the aircraft reaches cruising height, a smoker's ability to adapt to the slight fall in air pressure is very much reduced. Blood oxygen levels sink to significantly low levels. The body cannot store oxygen and it reacts rapidly if blood oxygen levels fall too low. Oxygen deficiency (called hypoxia) affects the brain, causing intense fatigue, dizziness, nausea, and lethargy, and repeated yawning is a sign of it. A heavy smoker really needs supplementary oxygen in-flight. If you are a heavy smoker:

- **Think ahead** and try to cut down during the days before a long-haul flight. The short pre-flight exercise programme on pages 30–31 will really help.
- **Try nicotine patches** to discourage yourself from smoking at all during the twenty-four hours before the flight.
- **Oxygen bars**, popular for some time in Tokyo, have opened in other world capitals, including London (at Harvey Nichols, a department store in Knightsbridge). You buy a mask, plug it into a unit, and breathe in lungfuls of pure oxygen. They are exactly what a smoker needs to boost blood oxygen levels before checking into an international airport for a long-haul flight.
- **Do not smoke in-flight**, even if the airline permits it. Not only are you in danger of developing hypoxia, but you release carbon monoxide into the cabin air, which reduces the blood oxygen levels of other passengers. Nicotine and other particles in smoke are removed by the air-conditioning system, but carbon monoxide is a gas, so the filters cannot remove it.

Divers

Flying at high altitude is like diving in reverse – pilots of jet fighters who climb very high very fast can get (aviator's) decompression sickness. The air pressure in a passenger jet is much too low for this to happen, but it can affect anyone who has been sub-aqua diving shortly before flying long-haul, and it can be fatal.

Decompression sickness is a condition in which nitrogen dissolved in the body tissues becomes gaseous and forms bubbles, which may circulate in the blood. Pain in the joints is a classic symptom, caused by nitrogen gas bubbles inside the joints. Tolerance is affected by ill-health, alcohol, smoking, drugs, being cold, and hypoxia (oxygen deprivation). People in their late teens and twenties, obese people, and those who have suffered a previous episode may have reduced tolerance, and some people are especially susceptible to decompression sickness. Divers should:

- **Not fly on the same day as a dive.** As a rule of thumb, leave forty-eight hours between a dive to depths greater than 10 metres (33 feet) and boarding the aircraft home.
- **Refer to reliable publications** for more precise technical information on time intervals between diving and flying. Those published by the US Federal Aviation Administration, the British Royal Navy, and the Undersea and Hyperbaric Medicine Society are detailed and dependable.

Climb and descent

Everyone is affected to varying degrees by the steady changes in air pressure as the aircraft climbs after take-off and descends towards landing. Passenger jets change altitude very slowly in a stepped pattern, taking an hour to reach cruising height or ground level, to minimize the effects on passengers. The ears are commonly affected, although any discomfort is quickly cleared simply by swallowing every so often as the aircraft climbs or descends. People who rarely fly may not know this, however.

The middle part of the ear has cavities filled with air. When the aircraft climbs, the pressure of the surrounding air falls, leaving the air in the ear cavities at a higher pressure. As the pressure difference increases with altitude, air suddenly escapes along the Eustachian tubes leading from the middle ear to the area just behind the nose, making popping noises. This happens automatically, and it is disconcerting if you don't know why.

The same thing happens in reverse as the aircraft descends for landing: the pressure of the surrounding air falls, so the air in the ear cavities is at a lower pressure. It is harder for air to enter the middle ear than to leave it, and the change in pressure causes the delicate ear drum to bulge inwards. This is uncomfortable, and the trick is to swallow repeatedly. Swallowing opens the Eustachian tubes so that air can flow into the middle ear. It can take a while for the pressure in the ears to equal the outside air pressure, and the ears can sometimes feel a little blocked for as long as an hour or so after landing.

Older children can be told to swallow, and young children can be given a hard sweet to suck so they swallow automatically when descending. Infants should be fed so that they suck and swallow, or given a rubber dummy or a finger to suck. They often cry, which does the trick.

Swallowing is necessary because unequal pressure in the ears causes the ear drum to bulge outwards during a climb and inwards during descent. This can become very painful if it isn't relieved, and in extreme situations the ear drum may be damaged, or burst, and the hearing can be affected. Bear in mind that the Eustachian tube often becomes blocked if you have a heavy cold. This is one of several good reasons why you should not fly if you have a cold. Another is that it releases millions of viruses into the cabin atmosphere and they can infect people seated around you. Sometimes, however, the tissues remain swollen after infection has passed. Inhalants, decongestants, gargling and all the other remedies for blocked sinuses (see below) will help clear blocked Eustachian tubes.

- **Valsalva manoeuvre**: if your ears hurt and you seem unable to clear them, this exercise will open the Eustachian tubes, but you must do it very gently: close your lips quite firmly, and hold both nostrils closed with the fingers of one hand. Blow air gently but firmly out between your lips while keeping your lips closed as though blowing, to increase the pressure in your mouth. This is like stifling a sneeze. Repeat as the aircraft continues to climb or descend and you feel discomfort increase in your ears.

● earplanes® are a kind of ear plug with a filter to regulate air pressure. They also screen out noise. They are available – for children and for adults – from pharmacists.

Blocked sinuses

The sinuses are air-filled cavities located around the nose. As the aircraft climbs, the air expands, and escapes through a tube leading into the nose. If any sinus is blocked, the air will be trapped and will press on the surrounding tissues as it expands. This causes sharp pain in the cheeks, forehead, or inside the head, and it makes the eyes water. In extreme cases surrounding blood vessels may be affected, and you might suddenly have a nose bleed during the flight or within twenty-four hours after you land, which may be very severe.

If you have a cold, the sinuses become inflamed and blocked by excess mucus. This is a third reason why you should never fly with a cold or a sinus infection (see pages 126–7, **Climb and descent**). If you have hay fever, however, you may find that the symptoms improve during a long-distance flight, because the air-filtration systems are very effective in removing pollen and other irritants in the air which cause a reaction. They also filter the air constantly, so pollen grains shed into the air from passengers' clothes as they move about the aircraft are constantly being filtered out.

If your sinuses remain blocked after a cold or an infection, try to clear them over a period of two or three days before your trip so that you can breathe easily in-flight. The following remedies will help:

- **Inhalants** such as Karvol (available over the counter in the UK) can be sprinkled on a pillow before you sleep or dissolved in hot water and inhaled. Karvol contains menthol and essential oils of the thyme plant, but aromatherapy oils containing eucalyptus or peppermint will also clear congestion.

- **A decongestant spray** such as Beconase may be necessary if you have hay fever or rhinitis, which inflame the mucous membranes of the nose and sinuses. It is fast-acting, so it can be used to clear the sinuses when you board the aircraft or as it starts its descent. Beconase contains steroid hormones, so check with a physician before using it.

- **Alternative therapists** recommend a daily dose of 500 mg of vitamin C combined with bioflavanoids to unblock a congested nose; and 200–500 mg supplements of pantothenic acid with vitamin B complex to relieve hay fever symptoms.

- **Aromatherapists** recommend packing a small bottle containing one drop of essential oil of lavender suspended in 5 millilitres of carrier oil or lotion, or one drop of essential oil of inula diluted in 5 ml of jojoba or sweet almond oil, and using the mixture to massage either side of the nose. Rest your head back against the seat and massage for about one minute.

● Gargling with a mouthwash or a drop of lemon juice in water will clear congestion from the frontal sinuses, which cannot be reached by massage, and will bring instant relief if your nose is blocked because you have been in a smoky atmosphere. You can usually find a washroom to gargle in, but do not use the hand-washing water in an aircraft lavatory for gargling. Some passenger jets have a drinking tap outside the washrooms.

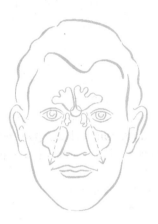

This illustration shows the sinuses or air cavities around the nose. A yoga exercise to relieve congestion is to stroke downwards using the middle finger of each hand, from just below the inner corner of each eye to the corners of the mouth, as indicated by the arrows. Stroke gently, several times in succession, and repeat the stroking often.

Expanding air

The body has many air-filled cavities, and during a climb the gas in these cavities expands. The expansion continues as you cruise in a cabin pressurized at a lower level than you are used to.

■ **Toothache** is very occasionally caused by expansion of air in a bad tooth as an aircraft ascends. It can also be caused in an old filling, but trapped air is rarely a problem in modern fillings. Regular dental checkups are the best preventive measure. Taking an analgesic is the only treatment while in flight.

■ **Stomach pain** during flight is often caused by the expansion of gas in the stomach or the intestines. This is normally only mildly uncomfortable and the gas escapes naturally as it expands, but if you have any infection of the stomach or intestines, the natural expansion may cause fairly sharp pain. Trapped gas causes no damage and the following measures will prevent and/or relieve it:

● **Don't** eat a very large meal during the twenty-four hours before a flight.
● **Don't** eat gas-forming foods, such as peas, beans, cauliflower, cabbage, cereals containing high quantities of bran, cheese, soya, and alcohol, or large quantities of biscuits or yeast bread.
● **Don't** drink carbonated soft drinks or sparkling mineral water.
● **Don't** chew gum: it makes you swallow air.
● **Eat and drink** slowly and chew food adequately.

- **The Hay diet** recommends not mixing protein and carbohydrate at the same meal.
- **Eat fruit** before meals, not with other foods or as a dessert.
- **Pack** a proprietary remedy for trapped wind in your hand luggage. They are advertised widely and sold over the counter by pharmacists.
- **Charcoal tablets** absorb gas and give immediate relief from pain and also from possible embarrassment.

HIGH-ALTITUDE FLYING

Do jets really need to fly so high? Why don't they fly at 1,500 kilometres (5,000 feet), say, so that pressurization, with all its health problems, is unnecessary? There are several answers, but the main reason is that modern airframes and engines operate more efficiently at higher altitudes where air resistance is low, and they are more economical on fuel. Low-level flying is dangerous, especially for an intercontinental jet cruising at about 885 kilometres (600 miles) an hour. Many of the Earth's natural features reach far higher than 1,500 kilometres (5,000 feet): the peak of Mount Everest is 8,848 metres (29,028 feet) above sea level, and La Paz, the capital of Bolivia, is 3,631 metres (11,916 feet) up. And aircraft flying at low altitudes are buffeted by extreme weather. Commercial jets fly in smoother and safer conditions at 10,700 metres (35,000 feet), above the worst of it, and supersonic jets, flying at even more exalted altitudes, look right down on it, thunderclouds and all.

Nevertheless, the argument about flying altitudes and cabin pressure never dies away, and in recent years some respected aviation organizations have revived it. The Air Transport Medicine Association recommends that the next generation of megajets should maintain a cabin altitude close to sea level. This view may gain more support if the results of research carried out in November 2000 are verified. Norwegian medical researchers reported an increase in the formation of blood clots in the deep veins of the legs in long-haul passengers shortly after the aircraft they were travelling in gained altitude.

CHAPTER SIX
The Cabin Environment

When it comes to regulations governing passenger aircraft, safety is the priority. Strict regulations require aircraft to have more than one source of fresh air to ensure a minimum supply, should one fail. There are rules requiring aircraft to carry emergency oxygen, which must be supplied to passengers if cabin air pressure falls below the equivalent of 3,000 metres (10,000 feet), and guidelines govern the proportions of gases circulating in the cabin air. But regulations aimed at providing passenger comfort are vague: ventilation should give 'reasonable' passenger comfort. Yet the freshness, humidity and temperature of the air in an aircraft cabin has a profound effect on the health and comfort of passengers who have to breathe it for eight hours or more. This chapter explains how an aircraft's internal air supply is generated and distributed through the fuselage, and it answers some frequently asked questions about cabin air supply and quality.

Where does the cabin air come from?

The supply of air for passengers and crew is fresh air drawn from the atmosphere outside the aircraft. Turbofan engines work by drawing in air and compressing it. Compression heats the air so that it sets the great fans that drive the engines in motion. Some of the compressed air, which is biologically sterile, is drawn off, cooled, adjusted to the required cabin pressure (see Chapter 5) and directed to air-conditioning packs which fine-tune it and distribute it to the flight deck and the cabins. Some is also used for necessary flying operations, such as de-icing the wings and fuelling the operating pumps for the hydraulic systems.

How much air does everyone get?

If the air in the cabin feels stuffy, passengers worry that they are not getting enough to breathe, but this worry is always unfounded. An adult sitting relatively still breathes approximately 6.8 litres (0.24 cubic feet) of air per minute at the standard cabin altitude. The need for air increases with activity, so cabin staff who are hurrying to serve meals are using about 18 litres (0.64 cubic feet) of air per minute, and if you had to run through the terminal to check in on time you could have been breathing as much as 100 litres (3.53 cubic feet) of air per minute.

This is not very much, aircraft engineers always point out, by comparison with the quantity of air available to passengers. Aircraft differ in the amount of air supplied, but the average air supply per passenger is 566 litres (20 cubic feet) a minute at the normal air pressure. This is more than thirty times the amount needed for normal respiration.

It is important to stress that these are averages, however, and that although the flow of air is more or less constant throughout the aircraft, the air flow per person is always reduced in economy class, because high-density seating means that more people are breathing the air flowing into that area.

Is anything added to or taken out of the air passengers breathe?

Air is made up of several gases: oxygen, carbon dioxide, nitrogen, and traces of other gases such as ozone. For air to be breathable it must contain roughly the same proportions of these gases as the air on the ground.

■ **Oxygen:** the air-conditioning systems do not change the proportion of oxygen in the air, which remains at 21 per cent, as at ground level. Everyone will have enough as long as the air pressure in the cabin is maintained at a level that enables the lungs to absorb enough oxygen with each breath (see pages 118–123).

■ **Carbon dioxide:** although this gas is thought of as a waste product because we breathe it out, carbon dioxide is essential to life. Its presence stimulates the breathing centres in the brain to regulate the rate and depth of each breath. It is harmful only when there is too much carbon dioxide in the air we breathe. The outside air at sea level contains about 0.03 per cent of carbon dioxide; indoors, where there are people breathing small amounts of carbon dioxide into the air, the concentrations are much higher. The maximum concentration of carbon dioxide permitted inside an aircraft cabin has been set by the regulatory authorities at 0.5 per cent. The ventilation system constantly removes it as it extracts the used cabin air, dumping it outside the aircraft while replacing it with fresh air from outside. The rate of dilution and removal of carbon dioxide therefore depends on the rate at which fresh air flows into and out of the cabin, but the level of carbon dioxide in a cabin with a full load of passengers is normally kept at 0.1 per cent or roughly four times the normal level in outside air at sea level.

The dry ice that chills food in the galley is frozen carbon dioxide. So that it will not contaminate the air when it vaporizes, and also to prevent strong food smells from pervading the cabin, the galleys have their own air-extraction system, separate from the cabin.

The slightly raised carbon dioxide levels are believed by physicians not to be harmful, since people have lived in air containing five to ten times the normal aircraft cabin levels for several weeks without experiencing any known ill-effects. Cabin staff appear not to experience ill-effects from constantly breathing cabin air. However, the carbon dioxide levels have generated some controversy.

Extra carbon dioxide was released into the air supply of many buildings in recirculated air systems introduced during the 1980s. It is thought to have contributed to 'sick building syndrome', which seemed to disappear from many buildings when fresh air ventilation was reintroduced. People are concerned that a 'sick aircraft syndrome' may be prevalent in high-flying, long-haul aircraft, perhaps caused by higher carbon dioxide levels in recirculated air.

■ **Ozone**: at high altitudes the air contains much higher levels of ozone than at ground level, especially over the Poles, and these levels change with the seasons. Aircraft sometimes pass through plumes of ozone which extend down to about 7,600 metres (25,000 feet). Ozone is a harmful chemical which in large enough concentrations causes dryness of the eyes and throat and difficulty breathing. Airworthiness authorities require that its concentrations in the cabin air never exceed the safe level of around 0.1 parts per million. To meet their requirements airlines can route passenger aircraft through zones with low ozone concentrations or install a catalytic ozone converter at the point where air is drawn in via the engine compressors. However, when aircraft not fitted with catalytic converters fly through ozone plumes, ozone concentrations in the air rise above recommended levels and cause minor symptoms in some passengers.

■ **Pesticides**: while an aircraft is on the ground before take-off, during a stopover, or after landing it is possible for insects to fly or crawl in. A recent check at one major airport found as many as five mosquitos in the cabins of aircraft just landed from areas where malaria occurs. World Health Authority regulations require all flights to be disinsected with pesticides before arriving at and/or departing from certain destinations. Aerosols may be sprayed in the cabin and lockers before anyone boards, and into the flight deck, cabin and holds after the doors are closed just before departure, or they may be sprayed into the cabin about an hour before landing. Food preparation surfaces may also be wiped over with an insecticide.

Many passengers hate this, some passenger health pressure groups question it, and the World Health

Organization is currently researching it. Meanwhile legal actions alleging harm from pesticide exposure are pending in the USA. The pesticides used are mainly pyrethroids, chosen because their toxic effects are minimal. No cases of ill-health caused by disinsection procedures are said to have occurred in the UK. Nevertheless several passengers who had been subjected to cabin spraying have complained that it has aggravated their asthma. It may be reassuring to know that after take-off the air-conditioning packs and extraction fans quickly clear residues from the air; and that if it occurs in the hour before landing, you will soon be able to get into fresh air.

Things you can do:
- To avoid the possibility of ozone contamination, all you can do is try to avoid flights that pass over the Poles. If you experience dry eyes or throat which you suspect may be caused by unsafe levels of ozone, try to find out from the cabin crew if the aircraft is fitted with a catalytic converter. You may be reassured, dry eyes and throat are also symptoms of dehydration (see pages 146–48) and can be relieved.
- You can express your views about carbon dioxide and ozone levels in cabin air, and disinsection procedures by writing to the airlines and to some of the organizations listed on pages 196–200 stating your misgivings and objections.

Does everyone in the aircraft breathe the same air?

All the air circulating through a passenger jet is drawn from outside. It circulates around the cabin, then 50–60 per cent of it is extracted by a fan and dumped overboard, and the remaining 40–50 per cent is filtered, mixed with fresh air from outside, and circulated. So each passenger receives on average 283 litres (10 cubic feet) per minute of fresh air mixed with a roughly equal amount of recirculated air. Airlines have different practices, however. On the Airbuses the proportion is 340 litres (12 cubic feet) per minute of fresh air and 227 litres (8 cubic feet) per minute of recirculated air per passenger.

For safety reasons, in many aircraft the flight deck has its own air supply, separate from the cabin. The Joint (i.e. European) Airworthiness Authority requires that the flight deck should receive air from a separate air-conditioning unit to that used in the cabins, and that it should be fresh air, not recirculated air. It has so far proved impracticable to implement this resolution. Air in the washrooms and toilets, as well as in the galleys, is continually extracted through separate vents and exited from the aircraft, so air from these areas is never recirculated and never comes into contact with cabin air.

Air from the engines is processed by two or three air-conditioning units before being directed into the cabin. In older aircraft it flows from front to back, and this tends to cause draughts in some spots and pools of stagnant air here and there. In modern aircraft it is flowed from ceiling to floor, over the occupants in flow patterns designed to maximize air movement and avoid draughts and stagnation.

Like pressurization, the environmental control systems in modern aircraft are fully automatic, but the crew can control the rate of airflow through the cabin, either by switching off one or more air-conditioning packs or, on the newer jets, by setting the rate of airflow through the packs to 'High', 'Medium', or 'Low'. It is essential that the flight crew should have this control: if passenger numbers are low, maximum air-conditioning may cause cold draughts in some cabin areas; and if the aircraft is full, maximum levels will make the main cabin too hot. Also, if one air-conditioning pack develops a fault, the other two need to function at a higher setting to maintain cabin air temperatures. Modern aircraft have the most sophisticated systems with adjustable settings so that airflow and temperature to different parts of the cabin can be fine-tuned. Some Airbus versions have up to six cabin zones.

All aircraft are different, and some have more efficient ventilation systems than others. For example, a feature article in *Time* magazine, 19 March 2001, cited confirmation by British Airways of apparent faults in the distribution of air through the new Boeing 777. The airline had received reports from air crews of passenger complaints, and had discovered still pockets of air forming at head height, causing nausea and dizziness in some passengers. The designers do not always get it right, and Boeing are consequently working on a programme of modifications for these new aircraft. In other aircraft it has been noted that the air-inlet grilles do not align properly with the seats.

Things you can do:

- Expect the air on a passenger jet to be a little stuffier than you would ideally like, especially in economy class when it is crowded. But if you think you are continually breathing really stale air, or you are much too hot or much too cold for, say, half an hour, tell a flight attendant. The air supply to your cabin zone may be adjustable from the flight deck.

- If there seems to be no change and you remain uncomfortable through a long flight, bear in mind that passengers' complaints resulted in action in the case of the Boeing 777. Write to the airline and to passenger health organizations (see pages 196–200) and explain your experience in detail.

How often is the air changed?

This necessarily varies between aircraft and airlines, because it is closely related to the rate of airflow through the cabin (see page 142, **Does everyone in the aircraft breathe the same air?**). The rate at which the air is extracted is computer-controlled, because it is part of the mechanism that keeps the aircraft interior pressurized to the required altitude. The typical airflow rate of 566 litres (20 cubic feet) per minute per passenger translates to a complete exchange of cabin air every every 4–6 minutes – or 10–15 times an hour per person. It is important to bear in mind that this is very much an average for the mix of 50 per cent fresh air plus 50 per cent filtered and recirculated air.

By comparison with the air in most people's homes and offices, cinemas, theatres, and even most hospitals, this air exchange rate is very high. And in fact, because only 50 per cent of the cabin air is recirculated, the throughflow of fresh air is even faster.

Can passengers control their air supply?

Not on most aircraft. Older aircraft had vents located above each passenger's head – similar to the nozzles usually found on tour buses and coaches – which could be turned on to direct a flow of cool air downwards. As an economy measure these have not been installed on modern generations of aircraft. However, in the opinion of many in the industry, this economy is at the expense of the passenger, as having some control over one's own immediate environment while travelling improves comfort.

Things you can do:
- If you think that a personal air supply would have improved the quality of your flight, write to the airline after the flight and say so. They will not be able

to install air nozzles ready for your next flight, but think of your letter as a contribution to a passenger campaign to have them reintroduced on new aircraft.

Humidity

Flying high above the clouds has the advantage that an aircraft is not tossed about in thunderstorms or struck by lightning while cruising, but it has the disadvantage that the air contains very little moisture. Humidity is expressed as a percentage of the maximum amount of water vapour air can hold: 100 per cent relative humidity (RH). After it has been compressed, which heats it to a high temperature, and passed through the air-conditioning packs, air flows into the cabin at 1 per cent relative humidity. By comparison, most buildings have a relative humidity of 30–70 per cent.

Down on the ground a low relative humidity rarely bothers anyone. Areas where rainfall is very sparse are as dry as any high-flying aircraft cabin, and millions of people live in hot, dry climates. On a long-distance flight, however, low humidity tends to affect health. Dry air causes dehydration, and that makes the blood more viscous, which may encourage traveller's DVT – the formation of blood clots in the deep veins of the legs (see Chapter 2). Dry air and a dry nose and throat are thought to increase the survival times of viruses that cause colds, flu, and related infections.

As a flight progresses, however, humidity is added to the atmosphere in many different ways: in a full cabin the passengers give off water vapour, and steam from food and drinks moistens the atmosphere. Recirculating 40–50 per cent of the cabin air keeps a high proportion of the moisture in the cabin, allowing humidity levels to rise as high as 20 per cent. Some airlines tried installing humidifiers, but this was not considered successful, because much higher humidity is likely to lead to water condensing on the wall panels and causing corrosion, possibly to vital aircraft structures and electrical systems. It is also absorbed by the furnishings, causing them to wear and adding to the weight of the aircraft. From an engineering point of view, low humidity in-flight is desirable.

Experiments carried out by the British Royal Air Force medical research organization demonstrated that people exposed to a relative humidity as low as 5 per cent for twenty-four hours did not suffer serious dehydration. The humidity in passenger aircraft during high-altitude cruising averages 10–15 per cent, but on a very long flight it falls as the destination approaches. People's tolerances differ and passengers report many uncomfortable symptoms: dry eyes, nose, mouth and skin, tiredness and headaches, and unusual thirst. And unaccustomed humidity levels can simply make you feel rotten. You cannot alter cabin humidity, but there are many simple measures you can take to prevent dehydration and relieve any discomforts caused by dry air.

Things you can do:

- **Drink plenty of water** in the few hours before boarding the aircraft, and drink a glass of water roughly once an hour during the flight.
- **Do not wear too many clothes** on board the aircraft, to reduce perspiration.
- **Wear glasses** instead of contact lenses, which may feel scratchy under dry conditions.
- **Fill a light plastic spray bottle** with water and spray a very fine mist in front of your face occasionally if your eyes start to prickle (take care not to spray your neighbours).
- **Hydrate your skin** with a moisturizer or a toner with a few drops of aloe vera juice or oil suspended in it.
- **Do not drink alcohol** while waiting for your flight or during the flight. It dehydrates and it increases urination.
- **Do not drink quantities of coffee** in the hours before the flight or during the flight. It dehydrates and it increases urination.
- **Do not smoke cigarettes** and avoid smoky areas before boarding the aircraft. Smoking dehydrates the skin.

Cabin temperature

Hot air bled from the engine compressor needs to be cooled before it can be circulated, so the airflow control and air-conditioning packs work together to bring a uniform temperature to all parts of the cabin. There are no rules governing cabin temperatures, but they are usually maintained at 22–24°C (70–75°F).

Temperature control is a delicate and complex operation involving many different factors. Before the passengers board, the air-conditioning is supplied by air bled from the APU (auxiliary power unit) to heat or cool the aircraft structure and furnishings. When the passengers board, each adds at least a 100 watt light bulb's worth of body heat to the cabin atmosphere. After take-off, with the passengers settled, this heat load reduces, but the heat of the sun may augment the internal temperature. Later, when the sun sets, this source of heat is lost.

The air-conditioning packs continually adjust for all these different factors. During the day, especially when the main cabin is crowded, their main function will be to cool the cabin, and at night and when passenger numbers are down, they will heat it. They are also programmed to maintain an even temperature from the flight deck and first- and business-class cabins, where very few people sit and the seats are widely spaced, to the main cabin where many people sit close together. Clearly, some seating areas may need to be cooled while others are simultaneously heated, so manual control enables fine-tuning of each cabin zone: air crew can add hot or cool air to the air emerging from the air-conditioning packs.

Inevitably, design faults and maintenance oversights will occasionally mean that cabin temperatures are too high or too low. The body is very sensitive to temperature changes, and a 'normal' temperature, however well maintained, will not suit every passenger: 70°F may be too hot for a fifty-one-year-old woman, but too cold for an eighty-year-old man. Normal reactions to temperature change, such as perspiring or gooseflesh, can make the environment feel insupportable during a long flight seated close up against other people. Tell a flight attendant if you feel too cold or too hot. Other passengers may be feeling the same, and the flight crew may be able to adjust the temperature to make you more comfortable. But be prepared to feel a little too hot or too cold at times during a long flight, and prepare in one of the following ways:

Things you can do:

- **Dress in layers** so you can peel off jackets and jumpers if you feel too hot, or don extra layers if you get cold. You lose 30 per cent of body heat from your head, so wear a cap or a headscarf.
- **Take spare lightweight underwear** to change into if you are hot. It will make you feel more comfortable.
- **Cool your skin** if you get too hot. Use a moisturizer or pack a small plastic spray bottle you can fill with cold water, and spray it around your face. Run your wrists under cold water in the washroom. Wring out a face cloth in cold water and sit with it draped over your forehead and temples, or around the back of your neck.
- **Drink refrigerated still water** if you are too hot.
- **Sitkari** is a hatha yoga exercise for cooling the body:

breathe out, purse your mouth, and let your tongue protrude slightly between your lips. Curl the sides of your tongue upwards towards the roof of your mouth so it forms a channel. Inhale slowly and deeply, drawing air along the channel in your tongue. Pull your tongue back, close your eyes, and hold your breath while counting slowly to thirty, then breathe out slowly through your nose. Repeat two or three times.

- **Keep doing the exercises** in Chapter 4. They will boost your circulation, warming your hands and feet if you are too cold.
- **Have a hot drink** if you are cold.

Breathing recirculated air

Aircraft engineers are mystified. Passengers have more air than they need, enough oxygen, a 50–60 per cent fresh air input every 2–3 minutes ... yet they complain and the press rants because a proportion of the cabin air is filtered and recirculated. Why?

Why recirculate?

Until the 1980s all cabin air on passenger jets was fresh air bled from the engines. Because it is heated to very high temperatures by the engine compressors, any micro-organisms are killed. It is then passed through heat exchangers to cool it to the required temperature and pressure, and through ozone converters, if fitted, then flowed through the cabin and extracted. Air crew and passengers who flew in the 1960s and 1970s look back with nostalgia to the days when cabins were fresh and aerated. More than one retired flight captain has reported noticing a deterioration in air quality on long-haul flights in recent years. Then fuel prices shot up and the airlines had to look for ways of saving costs.

Aircraft engines use a lot of fuel, and diverting some of the air they compress to ventilate the cabin has a cost in higher fuel consumption. Airbus Industrie engineers calculate that the air-conditioning raises fuel consumption by 3–4 per cent. Estimates of the cost of providing just 283 litres (10 cubic feet) of air per person per minute (half the usual airflow rate) are about US$60,000 per aircraft per year for an aircraft flying 3,000 hours per year, and the cost of kerosene taken to be US$1 per 4.55 litres (1 gallon). Reducing the amount of air taken from the engine compressor by 40–50 per cent and combining it with air taken from the cabin by recirculation fans cuts fuel costs and so keeps fares down.

From an engineer's point of view, recirculated air has many advantages apart from cost savings. It is already warm and can be flowed through cool areas to maintain even temperatures throughout the cabin. No moisture is lost in the recirculation process, so it maintains cabin humidity at a higher level than the exceptionally dry high-altitude fresh air from outside. And the two disadvantages of recirculating are easily overcome: carbon dioxide and other unwanted gases can be diluted by fresh air inputs and extracted; and any impurities that get into the air can be filtered out.

What do the filters remove?

Recirculating air involves passing some of the air extracted from the cabin through filters, usually one for each cabin zone. At the end of the 1980s, new high-efficiency particulate air filters (HEPA) were introduced and they were installed in the new generation of aircraft, notably the Airbus A340 series used on both medium- and long-haul routes. These filters maintain the highest achievable filtration rates – they are normally used in operating theatres. But even the circulation filters installed in the early 1980s achieve air cleanliness rates which far surpass those in homes and public buildings. Think of all the dust mites and the pollution caused by using 1,001 different chemical products to clean everything in your home.

What kinds of particles do these filters remove? Measurements in the 1980s showed that cigarette smoke was by far the worst pollutant of aircraft cabin air. Now that smoking is banned by many airlines, particles of nicotine and other chemicals associated with cigarette-smoking are trapped by the circulation filters, but they come almost exclusively from the clothes of smokers as they move around the cabin. Smoking has increased in many developing countries and in countries with fast-growing economies, however, and smoking is still permitted by some airlines from those areas.

Most of the particles in the cabin air come from passengers, whose clothes and bodies give off dust, pollen, seeds and spores, fibres, hairs, skin cells, dry-cleaning residues, and so on. The aircraft structure gives off particles from panels and decorative and furnishing materials and during disinsection procedures pesticides remain in the cabin air until they are removed by the air-conditioning system.

How effective are the filters?

The most startling result of tests carried out on filtered air is that if you take an absence of particles in the air to be an indication of its cleanliness, recirculated air is as fresh as fresh air taken from outside the aircraft at ground level. The HEPA filters trap particles as small as 0.3 thousandths of a millimetre in diameter (0.01 thousandths of an inch) with 99.95 per cent efficiency. This means that dust, tobacco particles, bacteria and all but the smallest viruses are removed from the circulating air, achieving hospital operating theatre purity levels. In fact the filters are so efficient that when the aircraft is on the ground and they are switched off, the fresh airport air that floods the cabin is considerably more polluted than the recirculated air it replaces. The air at cruising height has a higher purity than ground-level air, however, and the engine compressor does not contaminate the air with particles, so during cruising the contamination level of fresh and recirculated air tends to be equal.

However, the filters do not remove gases, such as carbon dioxide, or chemical compounds, such as those in cleaning products. They are dumped outside the aircraft in the air that is extracted. In exhaustive tests carried out during the late 1990s on operating Airbuses, more than fifty different chemical compounds were filtered out of the cabin air, but many of them were in negligible concentrations. The main ones were ethanole from alcoholic beverages, toluene and other aircraft fuel ingredients (which enter the air when the aircraft is on the ground), and formaldehyde and acetic acid from cleaning agents. Because they do not remove gases, the filters do not remove odours which can cause the air to seem stale.

Can the filters go wrong?

The November 2000 Report on Air Travel and Health published by the UK Government select committee (see page 194) notes that there appear to have been no independent tests of the efficiency of filters on the market. Tests like the one described above were carried out by aircraft manufacturers and airlines. Although one manufacturer reported that a filter would still continue working efficiently even if ruptured, there is clearly a need for independent assessment. Cabin crew sometimes report poor filter maintenance.

Equally seriously, the report noted that filters are

not inspected, monitored, or tested after installation. Suppliers of filters to aircraft manufacturers solemnly reported to the committee that yes, they can be faulty and they do go wrong. The report duly recommends regular in-flight monitoring of the efficiency of filters, especially in removing bacteria and viruses from the cabin atmosphere. Finally, the report suggests that the new and most effective HEPA filters, which are installed only on new generations of aircraft, should become standard on older aircraft still in service. These worries about the effectiveness of filters are echoed internationally, so the Air Travel and Health Report makes an important contribution to the dialogue. But it is now a case of wait and see.

If cabin air is as clean as operating theatre air, why does it always seem stale?

Operating theatres have one big advantage over aircraft cabins: structure, materials, furniture, and equipment are sterile, the patient is covered, and staff are shod, gowned, and masked in sterile coverings to keep to a minimum the level of contaminants being released into the air. And they are thoroughly scrubbed up with antibacterial soap so they are as sterile as humans can get. In that environment, the number of particles, bacteria and viruses, and the amount of body odour released into the air, are kept down to an absolute minimum.

In aircraft cabins, on the other hand, passengers and

crew are far from sterile, and a medley of continuous activity constantly fills the air with a fascinating variety of particles and aromas. It is significant that in particle measurement tests, the lowest counts are at night when most passengers sleep. During the day staff distribute food, producing odours and crumbs, alcoholic drinks, tea, and coffee, which evaporate into the air. They move up and down the cabin, raising dust. Everyone gets warm and perspires, and some people use after-shave, Cologne and perfume. People take their coats off, sit back on their seats, switch the video on, comb their hair, blow their noses, cough, and sneeze. All this keeps the filters very busy.

People do these things all over the aircraft, from the flight deck to the tail. In first class fewer people have more space to do them in, so although each first-class passenger generates roughly the same numbers of particles and smells, the air in the first-class cabin remains relatively fresh. In a full economy-class cabin large numbers of people use more air and generate more particles, heat and odour. If, as in some aircraft, the airflow is reduced in the main cabin, or the temperature is set too high, the air will be stale. So if you walk from first class or business class directly into a main cabin filled to capacity with passengers, the air quality may immediately strike you as less than fresh.

In addition, working aircraft systems give off strange smells. The UK's Royal Society for the Promotion of Health has recommended that research should be carried out into smells in passenger aircraft, similar to research into building smells.

Things you can do:

- If you book economy class, ask to sit at the end of the cabin closest to first class, where the air is likely to be marginally fresher.

- Be extra-thorough about personal hygiene: take a bath and wash your hair before the flight. Use anti-perspirants and a foot deodorant during the flight, and pack clean hosiery. Wear deodorizing insoles if you wear trainers. If you do all this, the air around you will smell fresher.

- Packing one or two clean clothes and changing into clean underwear or a freshly laundered shirt about halfway through the flight will make you feel cleaner and the air you breathe smell fresher.

- An alcohol-based Cologne or after-shave will freshen you and the air around you. Use it judiciously, however, because strong perfume may be unpleasant to neighbours. Choose something unobtrusive with a lemon base, or a diluted Eau-de-Cologne. If people seem to dislike it, do not use it again.

- Fan the air discreetly with a magazine for a few minutes if the air around you gets very stale. It will improve circulation in your immediate microclimate.

- If necessary, ask the cabin staff if the air circulation can be improved, or the temperature reduced. Write to the airline after the flight if nothing is done about it.

Can harmful chemicals from the engine get into the cabin air?

There is a large and very worrying question mark over this issue, and much more coordinated research is needed before this question can be satisfactorily answered. Apart from small amounts of chemicals escaping into the air from cabin furnishing and cleaning materials, harmful chemicals are only present in an aircraft in the form of lubricants, say, in the engines or the hydraulic systems, or air-conditioning coolants. These systems are sealed, so the chemicals have no contact with the outside air.

In recent years incidents have been reported in which passengers have noticed an unpleasant smell – the odour of unwashed socks is often recalled – which lasted for a few minutes. Following this, and occasionally for some time after the flight, passengers who experienced this smell have felt unwell, with headaches, nausea, even blackouts. These odours have been connected with incidents in which seals in engines or aircraft systems have developed faults, so that the lubricant oils have penetrated into the cabin air system. Alarm has been caused by the revelation that an organophosphate known as TOCP (tri-ortho-cresyl phosphate) has been used in aircraft fuels for years to reduce wear in the engines. Organophosphates are commonly used in agriculture, particularly in sheep dips, but they are highly controversial chemicals, because they can damage the brain and nervous system, causing twitching, and paralysing some parts of the body.

These are new concerns in aviation and very little has yet been done to investigate. As a result there is a surplus of scare stories circulating, but very little usable evidence. As this book goes to press, court cases alleging TOCP poisoning from cabin air are pending in the USA, brought by pilots who claim to have been affected. Pilots we have spoken to confirm that such leaks do occur. Immediately they sense a smell, a fine spray of oil in the air, or other signs of leakage, air crew disable the affected engine or air-conditioning pack to halt the leakage, and allow the air-filtration system to clear the air of residue and particles. Aircraft manufacturers and oil company executives questioned by the UK Government Science and Technology Committee in 2000 protested that the amounts of the chemical used in jet engine oils are so low as to be scarcely detectable, so that the oils are not classified as dangerous.

Doubts remain, and the Organophosphate Information Network (OPIN), the British Association of Air Line Pilots, and the International Association of Flight Attendants have all expressed concern and asked for steps to be taken to reduce the risk.

Things you can do:

● If apparent air contamination occurs while you are on board an aircraft, speak to a flight attendant immediately. Do not hesitate to do this: the flight crew know that passengers often detect problems before they are noticed on the flight deck, and the faster you let them know, the sooner they can take action.

- Follow the instructions given by flight attendants. You may be moved to another part of the aircraft where contamination has not occurred.

- Observe carefully what happens: remember any smell, any misting of the air, ask neighbours what they experienced, note the time the incident occurred, when it cleared, and what action was taken. Take careful notes. Ask questions and write down the answers.

- If you feel unwell, tell a flight attendant how you feel. The flight crew of all passenger jets have access to medical advice via radio.

- If you feel unwell later, after the aircraft lands, see a physician and explain what happened. You can ask to be seen by a medical officer at the airport, or be taken to a nearby accident and emergency centre.

- As soon as you have a chance, report the incident by writing to the Pesticide Action Network or any of the airline health organizations listed on pages 196–200.

Does recirculated air contain bacteria and other germs?

This is a big worry for many passengers: that bacteria and other germs released into the air by passengers coughing and sneezing are not expelled from the cabin by the extractor fans, but are circulated all around the cabin in recycled air, presumably increasing steadily in numbers. The engineers say no (see pages 154–5, **How effective are the filters?**) Below is one of the tests on which their answer is based.

Tests for microbes

Cabin air quality measurements carried out by Airbus Industrie in the late 1990s included counts of bacteria and other germs. Special devices capable of measuring small micro-organisms were installed on a working Airbus 310 and an Airbus 340, and air was allowed to flow through the devices at the rate of 50 litres (1.77 cubic feet) per minute for two minutes during flight. Analysis of the results found that:

- Most of the bacteria detected were harmless. (Many bacteria live in the human body, carrying out useful functions, such as aiding digestion in the gut.)
- No bacteria capable of causing serious infections were found. Very small concentrations were found of bacteria that cause skin infections, such as boils and styes.
- The overall levels of bacteria in the Airbus A310 cabin (with older, less efficient filters) were found to be only a little higher than the recommended germ concentration for operating theatres. In the Airbus A340 cabin (with new HEPA filters) the concentration was found to be equal to the recommended levels for operating theatres.

● The concentration of bacteria was higher in economy class (where there are large numbers of people) than in first class and business class (where passenger density is much lower). This demonstrates that the bacteria are being emitted by passengers in all cabin zones. If they were being recirculated in the filtered air, the concentrations would be roughly equal across all cabin zones.

Why do people get colds and flu on long-distance flights?

Everyone has a story: Mrs A developed a bad cough that turned into bronchitis. She was previously fit, so her doctor agreed that she must have picked up a virus in flight. On every recent flight, Mr B has caught a chest infection. Two days after flying home, Ms C was taken ill with a dreadful cold and is sure the air filters on her aircraft were not working properly.

There is a question mark here: colds and flu are transmitted by viruses, and all viruses are smaller than the smallest bacterium. The new HEPA filters remove all but the tiniest viruses, but people still worry that virus infections from passengers with colds and throat infections might be circulating around the cabin. Colds and flu are not just a feature of economy class: many frequent fliers in business class report that they always seem to have a cold.

There are many things to consider here and it is important to keep an open mind. First, there is a small window of possibility that on older aircraft with less efficient filtration systems, a smaller proportion of viruses is filtered out of the air than on newer aircraft with HEPA filters. Moreover, on old aircraft the air flows from nose to tail – from first and business class through the main cabin – whereas on the new aircraft it flows from the ceiling down to the floor. The risk of a virus infection on older aircraft might therefore be greater than on newer aircraft. But you have to set against this the fact that most viruses responsible for colds and flu normally live in the air for only a few minutes.

Infections are transmitted in several ways: through water droplets ejected into the air during coughing or sneezing, by touching an infected person, or by touching something an infected person has touched. We are all exposed to viruses all the time – you grab a shop door handle and you might grab hold of a billion viruses just deposited there by the last customer – but we do not always develop the disease they transmit. Whether we do so or not depends on several things: whether we have developed an immunity to that infection; whether the body's immune system is strong enough to fight it, how big a dose we picked up.

The verdict of health professionals who study this problem is that, although it is certainly possible to pick up a cold in an aircraft, the infection is least likely to be spread through recirculated cabin air. It is most likely to have come from contact with infected people, and that contact may not occur on the aircraft. A viral infection can take days to develop. You may be in close contact with infected people at work, at home, or out with friends. You may have briefly touched an infected person while travelling on a bus or a train on the way to the airport. The air terminal is crowded. You may pick up an infection while waiting in line to check in, or in a snack bar. And, of course, on the aircraft you may sit in economy class for eight hours or more just in front of a person with a cold, and you may pick up that person's infection.

All these possibilities will be repeated after you disembark. If your trip involves staying in a foreign country, be aware that you are more susceptible to infection while there. Every area has its complement of germs. If you live there you have a natural immunity to them, but you do not have immunity when you travel to new places. College physicians know that students studying away from home have more colds than usual during their first year since they do not have immunity to local bugs, and stress reduces their resistance. For similar reasons holidaymakers often go down with a cold while on holiday or just after coming back.

Laying the blame squarely for any infection you might pick up in-flight on broken filters or stale air is unhelpful. Cabin staff tend not to have a significantly higher proportion of colds than workers in other businesses. You need to consider all the possibilities, then work out how to avoid picking up a virus, or reduce the possibility of any you pick up developing into a full-blown infection. The best way is to relax and enjoy the flight. Do not become a victim to stress, which can undermine your natural ability to resist disease.

The first and most important consideration is the least likely to be observed, given the non-refundability of discounted airline tickets and the pressures on working people: if you get a cold or flu, do not travel. Not only are blocked ears and sinuses very uncomfortable in a pressurized environment but you are also likely to infect other passengers as you travel to the airport and on the aircraft.

Things you can do:

- Have a flu vaccination once a year (in September in the UK, otherwise check with a vaccination service). It will protect you against viruses currently circulating and you may find you do not get so much as a head cold all year long. Flu vaccinations may be available free of charge if you are over sixty. Younger people may have to pay, but the charge is small. The injection is suitable for anyone over six months of age and is effective immediately. It may be followed by a day or two of mild flu-like symptoms.
- Work and family problems, preparing to travel, and travelling are all very stressful and weaken the immune system. Try to prevent yourself from getting stressed (see pages 170–71).
- When travelling, try not to sit close to anyone who obviously has a cold. Ask to be moved to another seat.

- Never touch your eyes with your fingers without having first washed your hands carefully. Ophthalmologists warn that viral infection is transmitted very rapidly through the eyes.
- The mucous membranes in the nose and throat trap germs and viruses, but their efficiency is impaired in a dry atmosphere. Gargling with an antiseptic mouthwash will help clear infection from throat and sinuses and will moisten the mucous membranes. Also follow the suggestions listed under **Dehydration** (see pages 146–48).

Can you pick up serious illnesses, such as TB, in-flight?

Every health professional will confirm that cross-infection can always occur in a crowd, so infection is a risk that travellers on coaches, trains, ships and aircraft should be aware of and take every possible step to prevent.

Irresponsible press reports have demonstrably built up a fear that tuberculosis (TB) and perhaps other serious illnesses might be transmitted all over the cabin in recirculated air. There is more than one type of tuberculosis, but tuberculosis of the lung is caused by droplets spread by an infected person, usually through coughing. More than one case has been confirmed involving the transmission of infection in-flight, in which TB was transmitted to people sitting in seats close to the infected person. There is no evidence that TB bacteria were floating around in the cabin air and being breathed in by everyone. The people who subsequently showed signs of infection were sitting near the infected person for several hours. These conditions are unfortunately likely to produce cross-infection.

People infected with serious diseases are not permitted to fly under international health regulations, and airlines should refuse to carry them. But it is difficult to implement this rule because the incubation period for many diseases can be fairly long. People are often unaware that they have a disease, or the symptoms may not be evident to others. You cannot therefore know that you are sitting next to a person in the early stages of developing a disease, and there are no precautions you can take while in the aircraft. If a passenger is subsequently found to have had a communicable disease in-flight, the airlines will contact passengers thought to be at risk for testing.

Some passengers wear surgical face masks while travelling. A well-fitting mask might screen out infection if you sit directly in front of or beside an infected person (and it would lessen dehydration by preventing water vapour from your lungs from being dispersed into the air). However, it reduces the amount of oxygen you breathe in and increases the level of carbon dioxide in each breath. This might be unhealthy for some people, especially for those who tend to breathe shallowly when they fall asleep. Face masks are discouraged by some airlines.

Things you can do:

- Check whether you have been immunized against TB, and if not, have the BCG immunization. Tuberculosis is increasing world-wide and you can come into contact with it anywhere. Some strains are resistant to known drugs. A BCG immunization will be effective after six weeks, and one immunization will protect you for life.

- Check whether you have been immunized against poliomyelitus and tetanus, and if not, ask your physician for immunization or for a booster. Both are serious diseases and both occur widely.

- Children who need to travel should be immunized against diphtheria, which is increasing in some parts of the world.

- Make sure you take all precautions necessary to avoid infection with diseases prevalent in the areas where you are travelling. Check with a doctor specializing in travel health if you are unsure.

- While travelling and on board the aircraft pay scrupulous attention to personal hygiene. Wash your hands very thoroughly with soap and hot water after the lavatory and before meals. Take a small pack of Wet Wipes or similar products in case it is difficult to get out of your seat.

- Check for symptoms of illness for several weeks after your flight, and if you notice any, report them to your doctor.

Dealing with stress

On a long flight anxiety and stress are often the underlying reasons why people feel uncomfortable. They cause a dry mouth, sweating, alarming palpitations, headaches, and a sensation of not getting enough air. Some people get pins and needles in the hands and feet. Passengers sometimes faint on long-distance flights and those around them often assume that the air contains too much carbon dioxide or is otherwise contaminated. This is always possible, but it is significant that flight attendants have always been trained to look out for these symptoms: for passengers who just seem to look unwell – pale and a little dazed.

Flight attendants look first at the way the passenger is breathing. Very often breathing is rapid and some passengers seem to gasp for breath. These are symptoms of over-breathing or hyperventilation. It can occur in people with respiratory illnesses who are not getting enough oxygen, but it is also a response to anxiety. The breathing of a person under stress is often too deep or too shallow. These days flight attendants having to look after hundreds of people in a large aircraft may be too busy to notice this condition, but it can happen to us all and it is important to be aware.

What happens when you hyperventilate is that you breathe so deeply or so quickly that you breathe out too much carbon dioxide. Insufficient carbon dioxide dissolved in the blood makes your body too alkaline and causes all the symptoms noted above. If you recognize signs of over-breathing, the best thing to do is to breathe into a bag – a plastic bag or a paper bag will do – so that you rebreathe the carbon dioxide you are expelling. This quickly restores the oxygen balance of the blood and the brain responds by re-establishing a normal breathing rhythm.

Hyperventilation is uncomfortable, and if it is severe it will cause muscular spasm and loss of consciousness, so it is much better to be aware of how you feel. If you feel anxious and nervous, hot and headachy, or short of air, breathing fairly deeply and rhythmically for a few minutes will make you feel much better very quickly. The breathing exercises on pages 111–115 are designed to slow the breathing and, in so doing, to relax you. Here is an alternative exercise which you can use as first aid if you feel tense and your breathing rate and heartbeat seem a little too fast.

Things you can do:

- Close your mouth, make a fist with one hand and place your folded fingers and thumb against your mouth. Breathe in through the nose and exhale slowly through the mouth, forcing air through your closed lips and into your fist. Then breathe in again through your nose and repeat. Repeat the exercise four more times.
- Cool down: have a cool drink and rest back in your seat, perhaps with a wet cloth over your forehead.
- Gently massage your face (see page 104).

CHAPTER SEVEN
Eating and Drinking

Criticized by press and passengers for almost every aspect of the service they provide, including the meals they serve, airlines are rarely, if ever, praised for their success in delivering thousands of meals and beverages every year with few cases of food poisoning. There are estimated to be half a million people in the air at any time, and almost all will eat a meal in-flight. The food is prepared in airline kitchens where possible, but major airlines have to use contract caterers in distant countries. British Airways has reported serving more than 20 million meals a year from more than 150 kitchens and caterers located world-wide. So the fact that airlines maintain high catering standards in the face of increasing danger of contamination with salmonella, E-coli bacteria and other contaminants is a notable success. Meals served in-flight, if not what you would eat if you were at home, provide the kind of food it is advisable to eat on board an aircraft, and are generally nutritionally well balanced.

Guidelines for in-flight eating

It is important to eat and drink on a long flight. You need energy, and food and drink prevent dehydration, headaches, severe fatigue, and feelings of faintness. It is healthier to eat small meals and snacks than large meals – the quantities supplied by airlines is exactly right. Eating very large meals during the twenty-four hours before travelling increases the danger of a heart attack. Apart from avoiding gas-producing foods (see

Chapter 5 under **Expanding air**, page 131) there are no other rules to follow.

Cases of gastrointestinal infections clearly related to food served in-flight have occurred, however. It was as a result of a serious infection that affected half the passengers on a scheduled flight some years ago that the *Lancet*, the respected British medical journal, recommended serving the flight crew meals prepared in different kitchens from those where passengers' food is prepared, and cooked by a different chef. The World Health Organization recommended in 1997 that pilots should eat different dishes in hotels and restaurants before their flight, as well as on board the aircraft, so that a situation in which all crew members developed gastroenteritis would never arise.

It is as well to follow the WHO guidelines and be careful about food you eat in an airport, where food preparation and reheating standards may be poor. If you are nervous about food contamination, order a vegetarian meal instead of the standard meal, which usually contains meat. Most airlines cater for a wide range of diets. You have to order the type of meal you want when you book your ticket, and to be sure, reconfirm your order when you check in. Perhaps the safest food you can order is a vegan meal, which is based entirely on vegetables and fruit, and contains no meat, fish, shellfish, eggs, cheese or other dairy products. Here are a few guidelines to ensure bug-free eating:

● **Shellfish**: follow a longstanding tradition among air crew: do not eat shellfish of any kind during the twenty-four hours before flying, or, should they ever be served, during a flight.

- **Meat**: poultry and meat can harbour salmonella and E-coli bacteria, which cause intestinal infections and are widespread. Chicken and eggs are a particular risk. It may be best not to eat any meat while travelling.
- **Vegetables**: hot vegetable dishes are safer than meat-based meals, but avoid uncooked vegetables, eggs, mayonnaise, cheese and cream.
- **Soft cheeses** may harbour an organism that causes listeriosis, an infection resulting in inflammations in various parts of the body. It is especially dangerous to pregnant women and babies. It also occurs in poultry, meats, fish, shellfish and precooked foods. If you are pregnant, order a vegan meal when you book your ticket.
- **Hot drinks**: too much tea or coffee causes indigestion and has a dehydrating effect. Drink plenty of water while you are on board, and pack a few teabags containing fruit teas or other infusions which you particularly like.

Drinking water

Airlines usually supply bottled water for passengers to drink. However, it is sensible to take some bottled water with you to drink in case demand exceeds supply en route. In fact all on-board water should be drinking quality. All airports are required to have a supply of pure water. It must be palatable and clear, with no smell or colour. Before departure, large tanks on board passenger jets are filled from airport supplies by vehicles specially designed to carry drinking water.

Unfortunately, however, long-haul passenger aircraft cannot carry enough water for a round trip, so they need to top up overseas. At that point, quality control becomes hard to maintain. In recent years several articles have appeared in aviation trade magazines pointing out the now well-publicized fact that the demands on the world's water supplies are increasing in geometric proportion. While many airports serving the world's capitals and major industrial cities have been able to guarantee pure water supplies, this is becoming more and more difficult. In recent years smaller towns in the most advanced industrial countries have had trouble maintaining standards, and air crew sometimes uplift water from airports in developing countries where the required standards of purity are unachievable. Inevitably, therefore, there are reports of air crew having discovered that top-up supplies have been contaminated with harmful bacteria and other organisms.

To compound the problem, aircraft water systems are antiquated. Many otherwise state-of-the-art business jets are still fitted with water systems – and, indeed, with waste disposal systems – whose technology was state-of-the-art in the 1950s.

To prevent contamination of water and of on-board water tanks and pipes, World Health Organization recommendations call for the chlorination of all water supplies before they are distributed to aircraft. To make the water palatable, filters designed to neutralize the chlorine taste are fitted to the aircraft inlets, and neutralizing tablets are added to the supplies. No wonder pilots complain of the taste of on-board water! And no wonder flight attendants serve bottled water to crew! It is therefore depressing to learn from a recent US Food and Drug Administration report that one in eight bottles of mineral or natural spring water is contaminated.

Aircraft maintenance schedules provide for the sterilization of on-board water tanks and pipes every three months by flooding the system with chlorine-based additives, draining it out, and refilling the tanks with clean drinking water. But filters are no defence against micro-organisms, and any contamination occurring in mid-schedule will not be cleared until the next sterilization.

Like many issues of aviation health, the problem of water quality on passenger aircraft demands investigation. Anecdotes circulate of one corporate passenger having been hospitalized after drinking contaminated water aboard his company jet. Just one incident on an international passenger aircraft, where cabin water may be used to mix drinks, make coffee, and wash hands and dishes, could put the whole issue on the news pages.

New technology designed to overcome the problems is ready and waiting. One company has publicized the advantages of a revolutionary new sterilization system based on using ultraviolet light. As is often reported in studies of organisms living at the Poles beneath the hole in the ozone layer, ultraviolet light at high enough strengths can prevent organisms, including bacteria, viruses, and other biological contaminants, from reproducing. Manufacturers of the new technology claim that ultraviolet light destroys the ability of any micro-organisms in aircraft water supplies to contaminate the system, and produces better-tasting water. This system, which the company claims to have installed on many business jets, needs investigation, along with other new technologies on the market.

Things to do:

- Take some bottled water on a long flight and drink only bottled water supplied by the airline.
- Do not clean your teeth with running water from the washroom.
- Pack bactericidal soap in your hand luggage and use it to wash your hands very thoroughly if there is any possibility that soap in the washroom could have been used by other people. Non-bactericidal soap can harbour germs.

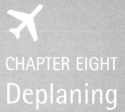

CHAPTER EIGHT
Deplaning

'Deplaning' is the name the aviation industry gives to the task of disembarking passengers with their luggage and escorting them through the maze of baggage collection, passport control and other necessary procedures. For passengers this part of the trip can be the worst, especially when a flight has been delayed. After several hours' travelling in economy class you can feel stiff, headachy, parched and dropping with fatigue, perhaps facing a long wait for bags. For nervous fliers, descent and landing are stressful phases of the flight and they disembark full of relief but bursting with undischarged tension.

As you disembark from the aircraft and pass into the terminal, make the most of the opportunity to walk with a spring. Towards the end of the flight you were probably feeling increasingly fatigued and less and less like squeezing past people to walk up and down the aircraft aisle, or running through an exercise routine one more time. Your blood circulation really could do with a boost and a brisk walk through to the baggage collection carousels is the best way of getting your muscle pumps going. If you have to stop and wait in line, lift your toes and heels and rotate each foot in turn.

The baggage collection bay may seem an odd place to exercise, but rather than sit on a trolley watching for your flight number to come up on a screen, give your whole body a much-deserved stretch. Stretching is something you can do quite discreetly even when standing wearing a coat and hat in a public place. Here are a few ideas:

Standing exercises

For all these exercises, stand with your legs roughly shoulder width apart, and relax your knees, just for stability.

Stretches

- Lift your spine from the sacrum at the base to the crown of your head. Then pull in the muscles of your lower abdomen and pull your pelvic floor muscles up. Hold briefly, then release. Rest and repeat two or three times.
- Clasp your elbows and twist your spine to the left and then to the right. Repeat two or three times.
- Clasp your hands behind your back, then straighten your arms and lift them up behind your back, bending forwards as you do so.

Shoulder roll

People naturally exercise their shoulders after a long period sitting still, by lifting and lowering them and moving them forwards and back. Do this exercise leaning back against a wall.

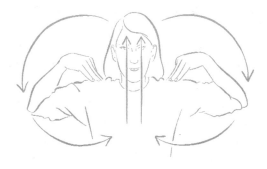

- Place your fingertips on your shoulders, breathe in, counting to three, then breathe out slowly, counting to six, while you push your feet down against the floor. Now slowly circle your elbows forwards until they almost touch, then up level with your ears, then back and down. Repeat. Then circle them in the opposite direction, moving them down, back, up, and forwards. Repeat and rest.

Circulation-booster

You may need to steady yourself with one hand against a wall for this exercise.

- Lift your heels and rise to balance on your forefeet, stretching your ankles, then lower your heels to the floor. Repeat two or three times.
- Kick your left leg forwards with the foot bent up. Repeat with your right leg. Then kick your left leg with the toes pointing forwards. Repeat with your right leg. Repeat two or three times.

Post-flight checks

The baggage collection bay is a good place to run a quick check for any symptoms of traveller's DVT. Is one ankle very swollen? Do you notice any pain in a calf or a thigh? Check through the list of symptoms on pages 50–52. If you have any doubts at all, contact a clerk for the airline from which you bought your ticket and ask to see a medical officer at the airport very urgently. If necessary, dial an emergency number and ask for an ambulance to take you to hospital. Remember to explain to the airport or hospital clerk, the medical officer or the physician that you have just disembarked from a flight and say that you think you have symptoms of a blood clot in the leg veins.

Symptoms of traveller's DVT can appear up to four weeks after a flight, so make those checks part of your daily routine for the next month. If you book a massage during this period, explain that you have been on a long-haul flight and ask the masseur not to work on your legs. Deep massage could dislodge a blood clot.

Checking for infections

People occasionally pick up an infection while abroad, so it is important to watch for the following symptoms and report them to your physician. Always say what country or countries you visited and when. Bear in mind that symptoms can appear months after your trip, so keep these checks up for six months after your return.

- Persistent stomach pains and diarrhoea: you could have picked up a bug which may need appropriate medication to clear it up.
- Flu-like symptoms with diarrhoea, a cough, a skin rash and pain in the muscles or joints: these symptoms need urgent investigation if you have visited a country where malaria is a danger at the time of year when you visited.
- Breathing difficulties and coughing: could be symptoms of several illnesses, including TB and parasitic

illnesses, as well as a sign of pulmonary embolism resulting from traveller's DVT. Go immediately to a hospital accident and emergency department, explain that you have travelled by air and ask if you can have a check for blood clots in the veins.

Carrying your bags

Do not add sore muscles and over-stretched joints to the aches and pains you have picked up en route. Take care lifting a heavy bag or suitcase (see pages 64–5), and if you have to carry your bags any distance try to equalize the weight on both sides. Lifting a heavy bag in one hand drags you over to one side, affects your posture, and hurts your neck and shoulders. For the next flight take a bag with wheels.

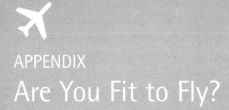

APPENDIX

Are You Fit to Fly?

Before booking a ticket for yourself and/or family or friends, check through this list. Some circumstances (such as advanced pregnancy) mean that airlines will not accept you as a passenger, usually for safety reasons. Others (such as lung disease) mean that flying would expose you to medical risks. Always bear in mind that flying imposes unusual stresses on the body, which may damage your health if you are not fit enough to withstand them.

Your health is your responsibility. The airlines reserve the right to refuse to carry anyone they consider unfit to fly, but they are usually happy to accept passengers who need special facilities, such as extra oxygen or wheelchair assistance. You must notify them in advance of any special condition and you may need written confirmation of your condition and needs from a physician. The airlines usually charge for providing these extra services. Many have a specialist medical officer who will answer queries.

The MEDIF form developed by IATA is invaluable for anyone with a medical problem who wishes to fly. The form is available from travel agents and from airlines. Part 1 of the form is completed by a physician, and Part 2 by you.

The following list is intended as a guide only. Check with a physician who specializes in aviation health before booking a flight if you fall into any of these categories or suffer any of the listed illnesses:

Infants and children

- Babies should not fly for two days after birth. Their lungs are not developed enough to withstand the reduced air pressure. Dehydration may also be a danger in the dry cabin air. Check with a paediatrician or a physician who specializes in aviation medicine if you intend to take a newborn child on a long flight in the first two weeks after birth.
- Children with ear problems should not fly.

Pregnant women

- Do not fly during the first trimester if you are prone to miscarriages.
- Most airlines will not allow expectant mothers to fly after the twenty-eighth week of pregnancy, but flying is considered safe until the end of the thirty-fifth week.

Lung and respiratory illnesses

As a rule of thumb, if you cannot walk 50 metres (55 yards) without getting out of breath, you will be affected by reduced cabin air pressure and will need supplementary oxygen.

- Severe asthma
- Bronchiectasis
- Chronic bronchitis
- Cor pulmonale

- Severe cystic fibrosis
- Emphysema
- Pneumothorax (collapsed lung)
- Pulmonary embolism (blood clot in the lung)
- Pulmonary fibrosis
- You should not fly for at least three weeks after major chest surgery.

Illnesses affecting the heart, blood vessels, and blood

As a rule of thumb, if you cannot walk 80 metres (88 yards) or climb a flight of 10–12 stairs without symptoms, you should not fly.

- Severe anaemia (you may need a blood transfusion before flying)
- Angina
- Coronary artery bypass
- Deep-vein thrombosis (history of blood clots in the legs)
- Heart failure
- Myocardial infarction (heart attack)
- Pacemaker
- Sickle cell haemoglobin C disease; sickle cell beta thalassaemia
- Stroke within the last three weeks
- Severe varicose veins
- You should not fly if you have recently injured either or both legs, or have had a leg operation.
- You should not fly during the twenty-four hours after donating blood.

Illnesses affecting the head and central nervous system

- Alzheimer's and other illnesses of which mental confusion is a symptom
- Epilepsy (you may need to increase medication for the flight)
- You should not fly if you have had a general anaesthetic in the last forty-eight hours.
- You should not fly if you recently fractured your skull or injured your head.
- **Ear:** you should not fly if you have otitis media or other severe ear infection, or if you have had a stapedectomy, or recent surgery to the middle ear.
- **Eye:** you should not fly if you have injured your eye or had eye surgery recently.
- **Nose:** you should not fly if you have a severe infection or inflammation affecting the sinuses.
- **Teeth:** you should not fly if you have had certain dental treatments in the last forty-eight hours. Consult your dentist.

Illness affecting the lower abdomen

You should not fly for two weeks after you have an operation to the abdomen.

- Recent haemorrhage in the intestines or bowel
- Incontinence

Other

- Cancer: check with your doctor if you suffer from cancer.
- Infectious diseases: you must not fly if you have an infectious disease, whether or not you are being treated for it: international regulations prohibit airlines from carrying infectious passengers. Flu and colds are infectious illnesses and it is better not to fly if you have them.
- Uncontrolled diabetes mellitus
- Divers: do not fly if you have been scuba-diving in the last forty-eight hours (see page 125).
- Psychiatric disorders (check with a psychiatrist)
- Terminal illness: you must check with your doctor and the airline before booking.

Medical insurance

It is unwise to fly without medical insurance. If you are taken ill in-flight, your aircraft may be diverted and you may be disembarked for medical treatment at the nearest airport. If you do not have medical insurance, you may have to pay for treatment and this can be costly. In some countries treatment may be refused if you cannot pay.

Medical insurance usually covers you for medical treatment in a foreign country for an illness that develops in flight. However, it is essential to ask the insurer to confirm that you would be covered if, for example, you developed traveller's DVT (deep-vein thrombosis) on the aircraft and had to have treatment at a foreign hospital. You must also read the policy carefully to be sure that this is written into it. If it is not, ask for confirmation in writing.

Insurers' conditions regarding insurance for people with medical complaints is complex and varied. You must contact the insurer in advance and declare your condition. If you are over sixty-five you have to pay a premium and you may obtain better terms by insuring through Age Concern or any other insurer who specializes in insuring older people.

For Europeans to claim free medical treatment in European countries of which they are not nationals, they need Form E111, obtainable from travel agents, consulates, and post offices. It must be filled in correctly, signed by your doctor, and copied.

You will need several copies of your insurance policy, Form E111, medical certificates, and, if you need treatment, of all bills, receipts, correspondence, and any forms you fill in.

FURTHER READING

House of Lords Select Committee on Science and Technology, *Air Travel and Health*, The Stationery Office Limited, November 2000.

An important report, available in public libraries in the UK. Sounds boring but makes fascinating reading. Full of useful explanations of how things work.

Ryan, Rob, *Stay Healthy Abroad*, Health Education Authority 1995.

A useful and readable guide to how to stay healthy once you reach your destination.

USEFUL ADDRESSES

Specialist medical treatment

Farnborough International Travel and Aviation Clinic
FITAC House,
159 Cove Road,
Farnborough,
Hampshire GU14 OHQ
Tel: [01252] 373755
Email: FITAC2000@aol.com

A specialist private clinic for aviation health problems. Contact for consultations, referrals, ECGs, blood tests, medicals, immunizations.

In-flight relief for medical conditions

Airogym Limited
Web: www.airogym.com
Exercise mat for in-flight use to improve circulation in the feet and legs, £7.99 by order from website.

The Back Shop
14 New Cavendish Street,
London W1G 8UW
Tel: [020] 7935 9120/9148/07000 BACKSHOP (international code: 44-2)
Fax: [020] 7224 1903 (international code: 44-2)
Email: info@thebackshop.co.uk
Web: www.thebackshop.co.uk
Dozens of devices for supporting the back suitable for in-flight use, including the Sitfit, the Stepfit, cervical rolls, posture pillows and a maternity belt. Mail order service.

No-Jet-Lag and Jet-Ease
Web: www.nojetlag.com and www.jetease.com
Contact the website for information about these homeopathic remedies plus listings of suppliers and stockists.

Air Transport Users Council (AUC)
CAA House, 45–59 Kingsway,
London WC2B 6TE
Tel: [020] 7240 6061 (international code: 44-2)
Fax: [020] 7240 7071 (international code: 44-2)
Web: www.auc.org.uk
Consumer watchdog for UK airline industry, established by UK Civil Aviation Authority to represent air passengers' interests and to back up the CAA in furthering passengers' interests to the authorities. Contact the AUC for advice on your rights and for complaints about conditions or treatment by cabin crew on air flights.

Aviation Health Institute (AHI)
8 King Edward Street,
Oxford OX1 4HL
Tel: [01865] 739 681 (international code: 44-1865)
Email: info@aviation-health.org
Web: www.aviation-health.org
A charity dedicated to investigating the effects of flying on passenger health and lobbying for improvement. Information, comment, research, action. VARDA is a support and lobbying organization for the families of victims of air travellers who died from traveller's DVT. Contact Ruth Christoffersen, Chair, at the AHI. Table of airline seat pitches published on AHI website. Online shop selling protective face masks, etc.

Civil Aviation Authority
Corporate Affairs Department,
Safety Regulation Group,
Aviation House,
Gatwick South,
Gatwick Airport,
West Sussex RH6 0YR
Tel: [01293] 567 171 (international code: 44-1293)
Fax: [01293] 573 999 (international code: 44-1293)
Email: aircraft: aircraft.reg@srg.co.uk
          medical: medicalweb@srg.caa.co.uk
Contact with complaints about any aspect of aircraft
safety, health and comfort, including seat pitch, cabin
air quality and pressurization.

Federal Aviation Administration,
Consumer Protection Division
US Department of Transportation,
Room 4107, C-75,
Washington DC 20590
Tel: 202 366 2220 (international code 1)
Safety & security hotline (toll-free in USA): 800 255
1111 (international code 1)
Email: airconsumer@ost.dot.gov
Contact for information or to register complaints
relating to travel on US-regulated airlines.

International Airline Passenger Association (IAPA)
PO Box 380,
Croydon,
Surrey CR9 2ZQ
Web: www.iapa.com
An international frequent airline passengers' club and lobbying association, established in 1960. Obtains discounts on a wide range of goods and services for members. The Office of Government and Industry Affairs formulates policies on safety, health, cabin environment and quality of airline service and lobbies appropriate companies and bodies world-wide for change. Check the website for details of your regional office.

National Radiological Protection Board
Chilton, Didcot,
Oxon OX11 0RQ
Tel: [01235] 831 600 (international code: 44-1235)
Fax: [01235] 833 891 (international code: 44-1235)
Email: nrpb@nrpb.org.uk
UK national organization to give advice and information on radiation hazards. Contact the NRPB if you have any questions or concerns about radiation levels in passenger aircraft.

Pesticide Action Network UK
Eurolink Centre,
49 Effra Road,
London SW2 1BZ
Tel: [020] 7274 8895 (international code: 44-2)
Fax: [020] 7274 9084 (international code: 44-2)
Email: admin@pan-uk.org
Web: www.pan-uk.org
An independent, non-profit-making organization working in the UK and globally to eliminate hazardous pesticides and other toxic chemicals in the environment. Contact them for information or to complain about the use of pesticides during a flight or about contamination with organophosphates. The organization will also advise on steps to safeguard your health if you have experienced a contamination incident on board an aircraft.

Royal Aeronautical Society
4 Hamilton Place,
London W1V 0BQ
Tel: [020] 7499 3515 (international code: 44-2)
Contact: Librarian
The RAeS has an excellent library with books and magazines on every aspect of aviation and a collection on aviation medicine. Open to non-members for a £15 daily fee.

World Health Organization (WHO)
Avenue Appia 20,
1211 Geneva 27,
Switzerland
Tel: 22 791 2111 (international code: 41)
Fax: 22 791 3111 (international code: 41)
Email: admin@who.int
Web: www.who.org

The WHO is an agency of the United Nations and responsible for preventing the spread of infectious disease through immunization and the restriction of travel of infected persons. Through its International Health Regulations it requires pesticides to be used for the disinsection of aircraft serving certain airports. Hit the WHO website for information about disinsection and for general travel advice. If you have concerns about disinsection procedures, contact the WHO at the above address, or contact your regional WHO office (addresses are listed on the WHO website and available at public libraries).

ACKNOWLEDGEMENTS

The authors would like to thank the following organizations and individuals for their help in compiling this book:

Virgin Atlantic Airways for their unstinting assistance in facilitating the testing of the exercises in first class, business class and economy class. Olwen Silvestri and other frequent fliers who tested the exercises for us on long-haul flights. Mr B. Riddle, Librarian at the Royal Aeronautical Society, for his invaluable help in tracking down sources of information. Captain J. L. Cox DFC, FRAeS and David East, aircraft engineer, for checking and correcting the technical information. Dr Staebler at his practice at 3A Ladbroke Road, London W11 3PA, for suggestions for homeopathic remedies.